THE FUTURE OF MEDICINE

THE FUTURE OF MEDICINE

Megatrends in Health Care That Will Improve Your Quality of Life

STEPHEN C. SCHIMPFF, MD, FACP

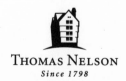

THOMAS NELSON
Since 1798

NASHVILLE   DALLAS   MEXICO CITY   RIO DE JANEIRO   BEIJING

Published in Nashville, Tennessee, by Thomas Nelson. Thomas Nelson is a trademark of Thomas Nelson, Inc.

Thomas Nelson, Inc. titles may be purchased in bulk for educational, business, fund-raising, or sales promotional use. For information, please e-mail SpecialMarkets@ThomasNelson.com.

The Future of Medicine provides information of a general nature, and readers are strongly cautioned to consult with a physician or other healthcare professional before engaging in any of the programs described herein. This book is not to be used as an alternative method for conditions requiring the services of a personal physician.

Information contained in this book or in any other publication, article, Web site, etc. should not be considered a substitute for consultation with a board-certified doctor to address individual medical needs. Individual facts and circumstances will determine the treatment that is most appropriate. *The Future of Medicine* Publisher and its Author, Stephen C. Schimpff, MD, disclaim any liability, loss, or damage that might result in the implementation of the contents of this book.

Library of Congress Cataloging-in-Publication Data

Schimpff, Stephen C., 1941–
  The future of medicine : megatrends in health care that will improve
your quality of life / Stephen C. Schimpff.
      p. cm.
  Includes bibliographical references.
  ISBN 13: 978-0-7852-2171-5 (hardcover)
  ISBN 10: 0-7852-2171-9 (hardcover)
  1. Medical innovations. 2. Medicine. 3. Medical care—Utilization.
I. Title.
RA418.5.M4S32 2007
610—dc22

                                        2007001646

Printed in the United States of America
07 08 09 10 QW 5 4 3 2 1

To Carol

My wife, helpmate, soul mate and partner for more than 44 years

Contents

Preface

This book had it origins in two parts. First, it began in my role at the University of Maryland Medical System where for eighteen years I was, successively, Executive Vice President and Chief Operating Officer, and then Chief Executive Officer of the Medical System's flagship institution, the University of Maryland Medical Center. I believed that the key to competitiveness was to recruit physician scientists who were at the cutting edge of new advances in medicine and to secure the most appropriate new technologies that would benefit our patients in their care. This meant being up-to-date on the advances in medicine and science so that the most appropriate decisions could be made about directions and technologies.

I was constantly talking to experts far and wide, attending meetings and symposia, and reading articles to stay up-to-date. Then came a request for me to give a talk on the "Future of Medicine" to a chamber of commerce group. They left the contents up to me. After some thought, I decided I did not want to focus on the many problems besetting medicine today, such as the appalling lack of insurance by more than 40 million Americans; the disparities of care among the rich and poor and among minorities; the excessive governmental regulations that sap all too much time from doctors, nurses, and pharmacists; the problems of individuals using the local emergency room as their primary care clinic; and the excessive rise in health care costs without concurrent improvements in basic health measures among the population.

All very important for sure, but I decided to focus on the tremendous and exciting advances that were being made—and rapidly—in the practice of medicine. In effect, this talk gave me the opportunity to synthesize my thinking about the directions our medical center needed to be taking.

To get better prepared, I interviewed many colleagues both at the University of Maryland Medical Center and at the National Institutes of Health where I was then a member of the Clinical Center Board of Governors. Very quickly, a set of "revolutions" in research and development emerged, such as genomics, stem cells, and technology advances that were having a decided impact on medical care or would continue to be in the not-too-distant future. These then became the basis for my presentation.

It was new for me to talk to lay groups, but it went well, and I was asked to come back with an update the following year. Others began asking me to give the same talk—Johns Hopkins classes in management, the University of Baltimore management classes, a national law firm, even an art group. I also used it frequently when meeting with groups of potential donors to the hospital. Each time, the talk was met with great interest and the Q&A period went well over the allotted time. Eventually, I began to think this material would be a useful book for lay persons interested in their own and their families' health. So after I retired, I decided to put these thoughts to paper. But medicine is moving fast, and I needed to update my materials and my thinking.

My process in researching this book has been to interview more than one hundred leaders in their fields. Some have been deans of medical schools or CEOs of academic hospitals, but most have been the physicians, scientists, engineers, and computer scientists who are at the forefront of medical advances. Although I had a written list of sequential questions to ask, in most cases, I began our interview with a very broad, open-ended question such as, "Tell me what you think will be the major advances in medical care over the next five to fifteen years."

This was usually enough to get each person going. Then I would listen and, based on what I heard, try to keep the person on track, or I would bring them back to address an issue mentioned but not yet clarified. In some interviews when I was seeking added information about a specific topic, I was more directive and narrow, such as asking, "Tell me what you think will be the major advances in stroke management and prevention in the years to come."

The material on patient safety was developed in a similar process and was also based on many interviews, this time with physicians, nurses, pharmacists, and hospital executives, along with leaders at major key organizations, such as the Joint Commission of Accreditation of Healthcare Organizations.

Everyone was very helpful and forthcoming. My next task was to find the threads of ideas that pulled all of these comments together. Being a "lumper" rather than a "splitter," I soon had culled the information down into a group of megatrends, and it is these megatrends that are the essence of this book. Have I missed some megatrends? For sure. And will some argue that I could have lumped things differently? Certainly. But these seemed to be the biggest trends, and they were magnified time and time again by so many of the people that I talked to. I hope you find them useful.

Introduction

When I was a child my mother told me about my grandfather and his medical practice. He grew up in mid–New York State on a farm. He and his father arose by 4:00 a.m., ate some bread and drank warm milk that had been left on the kitchen table the night before, and then headed for the barn to milk the cows, fork the hay, collect the eggs, and let the animals out to pasture before returning to the kitchen for breakfast. Then my grandfather was off to school. He graduated with the first class in the first high school in the area and went to Union College in Albany.

At some point, his mother became seriously ill, and he decided to become a physician, enrolling after graduation in Albany Medical College, a medical school that required a bachelor's degree before entry, which was still a rarity in those days in the 1890s. His mother died during his medical school years, but his father withheld the news for a while until exams were over; he didn't want his son to be distracted.

After medical school, my grandfather did an internship and then returned home to join another physician's practice in the adjoining town. Soon he married and he and my grandmother set out for Fishkill Landing, later to become Beacon, a small town on the Hudson River, about one hundred miles north of New York City. His office was in a room at the side of the house with a separate entrance off the large, wraparound porch that served as the waiting room. Basically, it was first come, first served until everyone had been seen. My grandmother served as receptionist, but her major role was to care for the family since her husband was so often called out. They had a phone, and it was constantly ringing with a request to see a sick family member.

Four children arrived during the course of seven years, my mother being the youngest. She often went with her father on house calls, first in a horse and buggy and later in a Model T Ford. She remembered his black bag, which carried all of his instruments plus many vials of medications. Families paid in cash—often literally pulled out from under the mattress—after he performed a delivery. Often the family or patient could not pay, at least not right away. But then in the fall, as the harvests came in, the local farmers would drop by with a bushel of apples or potatoes that would be left on the kitchen stoop.

The family lived comfortably in a modest home in a modest neighborhood and had enough that my mother was sent to a private girls' school and then to college. But certainly they were not rich nor were most physicians of that time. It was a noble profession with lots of personal kudos and a sense of satisfaction, but also with many late nights watching over a sick child or delivering a baby on the patient's kitchen table. Truth was, a doctor in those times could do very little to treat or cure anyone.

Medical school was mostly about becoming an expert diagnostician, one who could determine what was wrong and tell the patient and the family what the likely course of the disease would be. Diseases inevitably progressed because actual treatments were few and far between. The black bag contained mostly herbal extracts that did little, as well as morphine for pain and digitalis for heart ailments. Prescriptions were all essentially the same. Pharmacists compounded the prescriptions written in Latin, and placed them in bottles with a label that told how much to take but not what the medication actually contained, nor what it was supposed to do. It was a mystery—magic even—that was between the patient, the doctor, and the pharmacist. Sometimes it worked, mostly it didn't. Diseases simply had to run their course, as predicted by the physician.

Caring for and attending to the patient, recommended by the doctor but provided by family members, often made the most difference. Hospitals were uncommon and were mostly meant for the dying. But hospitals did have nurses who could give what was called supportive care—food, drink, cold baths to bring down a fever, and clean bedclothes after a high fever. A good nurse could help a person back to health. So my grandfather was anxious to see a hospital built in his town, and eventually one was, just across the street from his home. But mostly his skill and his value lay in his ability to interact with individuals, tell them what was wrong, and give them hope that they would be better over a course of time—or to help them and their family deal with the fatality that was bound to be.

He died in his mid-sixties in 1936 of a heart attack. He had lived just long enough to see a remarkable change begin in medicine—based on developing science. X-rays, which had been around since the early twentieth century, allowed a doctor to check for broken bones before setting and applying a cast. Chest X-rays revealed pneumonia, and barium for enemas let physicians look at the colon or even, if swallowed, the stomach. Insulin had been discovered in the 1920s and was just beginning to be used for a few people with diabetes.

After my grandfather's death, the first sulfa drug would dramatically shorten the course of many infections and even cure some usually fatal infections like meningitis. Penicillin was on its way. Laboratory medicine—with techniques to measure various substances in the blood, such as sugar levels or blood counts—made inroads in medical practice. And the major infections of his early practice years, typhoid and tuberculosis, for example, diminished as a result of good sanitation with water and sewers and pasteurization of milk. Some vaccines had made a big dent in diseases as well, such as those for small-pox and tetanus.[1]

So the paradigm of medicine was changing from one of "diagnose and predict outcome" to one of "diagnose and treat," a momentous change. This is the medicine that I grew up with during my years of practice, teaching, and research—one where science has been constantly uncovering new information and from it new approaches to treatment and cure. But the advances in treatment came with a cost to the patient in attention and care. Indeed, many say that medicine and physicians in particular have become "cold," that the caring of the past has been lost. To some degree that is true and it is a loss of great import and of great proportion.

Without excusing my colleagues who are in too much of a hurry to see the next patient, who do not have that "old-fashioned" rapport with their patients, who do not spend enough time to listen and to comfort, I would add that today's doctors can make almost everyone better to some degree and cure many. Hospitals are no longer for dying, but for complex, major operations such as heart bypass or valve replacement or kidney transplants; for treatment of cancer that would have killed earlier patients; for infusion of clot busting drugs to reverse the paralysis of a stroke; or for the repair of major trauma that in the past would have killed or maimed a patient for life.

Still, I hope that my grandfather's compassion and commitment to his patients was passed down to me via my mother and that my patients felt that I used those skills for their benefit during the years. I think that the loss of many of the skills of my grandfather's generation is sad, but I can also appreciate the benefits that medicine can give today.

The paradigm is changing once again. I believe it will soon change from "diagnose and treat" to "predict and prevent." The possibility exists to know what a person is predisposed to develop with time—heart disease, cancer, diabetes, and so on. With this knowledge, the physician of the not-too-distant future will be able to prescribe a defined approach to lifestyle changes, medications, or special devices that can alter the long-term course of diseases and even prevent their appearance. Prevention will also have a dramatic effect in reducing the costs of health care, now rapidly rising.

Predicting and preventing is a major theme of this book. But other themes are presented as well, such as engaging engineering and computer science to create imaging equipment that can peer into the body in noninvasive manners, yet create exquisite and detailed anatomic and metabolic images. Or to build devices that can measure the level of sugar in the patient's blood and then automatically administer the exact amount of insulin needed to a diabetic whose pancreas can no longer respond. Or to use the data from the imaging studies to set up a simulation of the needed operation that the surgeon will practice in advance, and then use that simulated, practiced product to program robots to assist the surgeon with the actual operation the next day—all to improve the outcome of the surgery and make it so much safer.

Information technology will be used to create an electronic medical record, one that can travel with you all the time and be available at a moment's notice no matter where you or your physician might be. This book is about the new drugs that are being developed, often with the aid of genomic information that gives the new drug a specific target to attack, resulting in more effective medications and much safer ones as well. It is about the resurgence of ancient methods of care such as acupuncture, which are having a rebirth of respectability in medical practice, along with proof of their efficacy for specific problems, such as the pain of osteoarthritis. Finally, it is about how each of us is still responsible for our own health and what we must do to preserve it.

One more element to these advances, I hope, is about how new technologies can actually bring the health care provider and the patient back together. We can use our advancing technology to "rehumanize" medicine—not the other way around. Technical advances need not mean dehumanizing medicine. We can do more today; we can cure more today and this will only advance further in the coming years. We don't want to go back to the past when there was little that could be specifically done.

We would certainly like to have *magnetic resonance imaging* (MRI) performed on our brain rather than undergo a lumbar puncture to extract some fluid for analysis. We would certainly prefer to have our gallbladder removed through the tiny incision of the laparoscope rather than a big incision. We would not want to go back to the days when ulcers were often treated with surgery rather than antibiotics to kill the causative germ. We are also learning that what we call diabetes in one person is not the same diabetes in another person. Each has his or her own disease and each needs care designed for him or her—personalized medicine.

So times are better, yet we—providers and patients alike—believe that the "golden age" of Marcus Welby is past. Providers feel overwhelmed with regulatory requirements that sap time away from patient contact; overwhelmed by the need to get permission from insurers who make their call centers slow to respond; burdened by the costs to engage clerks and billing agents rather than nurses to add value to the patient's experience; annoyed that our health care system does not pay for preventive care, many aspects of rehabilitation care, or even for time to just sit and talk about the totality of a person's life and how it affects his or her health and disease.

Yet we can hope that new technologies will make care more affordable, more accessible, and more personalized. We need to look at each new technology and determine if it can bring the provider back to a humane encounter with the patient. Technologies can radically alter the experience of medicine and hence the relationship between the patient and the provider—be that the doctor, nurse, pharmacist, or physical therapist. Health care providers went into medicine because in their hearts they want to be healers. The pendulum will swing away from regulations and the time-wasters so commonplace today, and the new technologies will help providers get back to being healers once again. As we develop more and more "personalized medicine," I believe we will once again come back to how medicine was practiced in the past.

But now, let us look at the future and examine some of the trends—I call them "megatrends"—that will change medical practice and hence your care dramatically over the next five to fifteen years. Some megatrends are the result of steady advances in biomedical and bioengineering science but many are truly transformational or disruptive—megatrends that will fundamentally alter the way medicine is practiced. I have divided them into sections. The first section chronicles the discoveries in the basic science laboratories that are bringing forth the advances of genomics, stem cells, and vaccines. The second is from the engineering and computer scientists who create tiny, powerful medical devices, incredible imaging equipment, new tools for the operating room, and the ability to digitize your medical record. These advances prompt a brief discussion of rising health care costs.

The third section is back to the future, as ancient healing practices are once again becoming not only popular but also being understood scientifically. And slowly but surely we in medicine are learning basic industry approaches to improving safety for all patients. Finally, I wrap up our discussion with what each of us needs to do to maintain this incredible body and mind we were given at birth. It is our responsibility, and if we treat them well, then the megatrends in medicine will be there to help when something does go wrong.

PART I

From the Biomedical Research Laboratories

Part I looks at the dramatic advances occurring as a result of basic scientific discoveries made in the biomedical research laboratories of the academic medical centers, the National Institutes of Health, and the pharmaceutical/biotechnology industry. These discoveries are the driving forces of genomics, stem cells, and vaccine developments that will be described and how they will create megatrends in the fundamental nature of how patients are cared for by their health care providers. We will see how the concept of personalized medicine can become a reality and how some of the basic paradigms of medical care will change, such as a change from today's "diagnose and treat" to tomorrow's "predict and prevent."

CHAPTER 1

Genomics—A New Era for Medicine

We have entered into a new era in medical care, the era of genomic medicine. In coming years, we will see an improved ability to diagnose a disease and even to predict diseases to come later in life. A much more accurate prognostication of what will happen as the disease progresses and how it responds to medications will be offered, and treatment will improve. Drug therapy will change so that new drugs will be more effective and much safer. Physicians will be able to select a drug based upon an individual patient's personal way of responding to that drug, both in terms of greater effectiveness and in terms of reduced side effects.

Even the foods we eat will be understood in terms of how they affect a specific individual. Vaccines will be "designed" for an individual patient who has, for example, a particular type of cancer that has been reduced but not totally eliminated. Finally, actual gene therapy—the introduction of a new gene to correct one that is diseased or will cause disease—will become commonplace, such as a true cure for sickle cell anemia or perhaps cystic fibrosis. Genomics will permeate all branches of medicine.

Medical practice changed dramatically in the middle of the last century. Earlier, a physician attempted to understand what disease was present so that he could tell the patient and family its likely outcome. Specific therapies were few and far between. Then medicine became a true science with an increasing understanding of the cellular and molecular mechanisms that underlie each illness. With that developing knowledge, doctors could begin to treat disease with greatly improved medicines, such as penicillin for infections, tPA for breaking up blood clots in a stroke or heart attack, and drugs like phenothiazides for serious mental illnesses like schizophrenia.

Doctors and patients both saw penicillin as a miracle drug when it first was used to treat serious pneumonias. I am still in wondrous amazement when I see a person with a stroke come to the emergency room unable to move his left side, only to watch him stand up and walk an hour later after receiving tPA. And the state mental hospitals—long used to "warehouse" individuals with chronic mental illnesses—have been eclipsed by the use of potent drug therapies that get people back home and enjoying life again.

But now we are entering a whole new era. The genomic era will allow for a change in your physician's basic approach, from one focused on detecting a disease and treating it, to one where she is focused on predicting a disease later in life and prescribing a preventive approach. (I use the pronoun *she* here to emphasize another major trend in medicine—today over 50 percent of medical school students are women.)

Consider Anna Blumenthal, a thirty-four-year-old single woman employed as a financial consultant with a major accounting firm in the mid-Atlantic area.[1] She began to have intermittent episodes of breathing difficulty and her doctor diagnosed asthma, a condition in which the smooth muscles around the airways deep inside the lungs begin to constrict, making it difficult to move air in and out and creating the characteristic wheeze during exhalation. Her doctor reviewed a variety of things she could do at home to reduce her chance of developing asthma attacks and gave her some preventive medications as well. He also gave her a prescription for an albuterol inhaler and told her to keep it handy for use in case of an asthma attack.

She followed her doctor's instructions, making some changes in her environment and taking the preventive medications regularly. However, at about two o'clock one morning, she woke up, struggling to breathe. Alone at night, it was scary. But she remembered the albuterol that was in her medicine closet. She had read the instructions before but now read them again.

Albuterol comes in a spray canister; you put your lips around a mouthpiece, press down on the canister, and out comes a measured amount of very fine spray. The idea is to press the canister while taking a deep breath in, so that the medicine will get deep into the lungs. Albuterol works because it interacts with a receptor on the lining of the airways of the lung, a receptor that can relax the smooth muscles that are causing the constriction. When albuterol finds that receptor, it breaks the action of the smooth muscle constriction. It doesn't cure the underlying cause that created the constriction in the first place, but it can turn the attack around in the short term. This receptor is the product of a specific gene that is part of our DNA. So we can say that our DNA directs the production of this receptor along our airways that will respond to albuterol.

Anna knew that after breathing in the albuterol she should begin to feel relief within a few minutes. She put the mouthpiece in, depressed the canister, breathed in the spray, and repeated it about a minute later, as directed. Then she waited, but nothing happened. Indeed, it was getting more difficult to breathe not less difficult. Now she really was scared because the promised relief had not arrived. Why? Because Anna is one of those rare people who are born with a gene that directs the production of a slightly different receptor on the lining of her airways, and this slightly different receptor does not respond to albuterol.

The middle of the night during an acute asthma attack is hardly the time to discover that you are among the unfortunate few. But for years physicians have been unable to predict which patients would not respond to albuterol. As a result of genomics, soon it will be possible to know who will not respond, so that an alternative medication can be prescribed and a long night of distress—and fright—can be avoided.

DNA and the Creation of Proteins

The genomics era began at the start of this century with the preliminary sequencing of the entire human genome, a task that was completed in 2003. What does this mean? How does it affect your medical care? A brief review of the structure and activity of DNA will be helpful before I attempt to answer these questions.

Left—DNA double helix; Right—Demonstrating the linkage of A to T and C to G
Courtesy Thomas Jemski, University of Maryland School of Medicine.

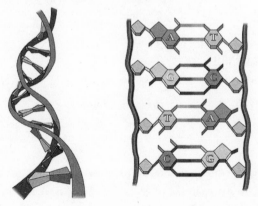

Deoxyribonucleic acid (DNA) is made up of molecules of four substances *(nucleotides)* that are named adenine (A), thymine (T), cytosine (C), and guanine

(G). For our purposes let's just use the letters A, T, C, and G. They are attached to a "backbone" of sugars and phosphate. DNA has two main jobs. One is to replicate itself and the other is to direct the production of proteins.

Replicating itself allows a copy of DNA to be created whenever a new cell is created. Proteins are critical cellular compounds that control a cell's basic functions and structure. DNA ultimately establishes what a cell is and what it does. Proteins, in turn, are made up of molecules called *amino acids* of which there are twenty types, all arranged in a specific sequence that is different for each protein. DNA directs the sequential arrangement of amino acids, a task accomplished by the arrangement of the A, T, C, and Gs of DNA.

Each and every cell has our entire DNA. Half of it comes from Mom and half comes from Dad. It's arranged in units *(chromosomes),* twenty-three from each side of our family for a total of forty-six. DNA is basically a long chain of those four letters A, T, C, and G. These four letters make up the genomic alphabet. They can be put together in groups of three that code for a specific amino acid.

For example, ACA is the code for the amino acid histidine, which is one of the twenty that make up proteins in the body. CAC is the code for threonine, another amino acid that makes up protein. These three-letter codes are called *codons,* and we can think of each of them as a "word" in our genetic dictionary. Consider a long chain of ACACACACACACAC, and so forth. This would be a code for alternating the amino acids histidine and threonine.

Dictionary of Genomics

BOOK—	Genome
CHAPTER—	Chromosome
PARAGRAPH—	Gene
WORD—	Codon (3-letter code, e.g., AAC)
LETTER—	Nucleotide (A, T, C, G, i.e., the four "letters" in the genetic alphabet)

A set of codons, which we can call the gene, is the blueprint for the structure of a protein. In my example of ACACACACAC, we are not making a true protein but an alternating chain of these two amino acids. The process goes like this: Our gene, which would be part of the entire strand of DNA, directs the creation of a related compound called mRNA (*messenger RNA*). The mRNA, which holds the same code,[2] travels to a part of the cell called the *ribosome;* a ribosome is basically a protein manufacturing factory. The ribosome takes the mRNA and follows the code, in this case alternating ACA, CAC, ACA, etc., and puts together the alternating amino acids histidine and threonine.

A real protein, such as insulin or hemoglobin, is made up of many different amino acids and usually is many hundreds of amino acids long. After it's manufactured by the ribosome, it "folds" into a complicated shape that might look like a ribbon sort of wiggled together on the floor after coming off a Christmas package. In fact, that shape is very specific and allows for the creation of an active site on the protein, which is the part of the protein that causes something to happen, such as relaxing the smooth muscles around the airways.

How much DNA do we have in each of our cells? If we were to "read" one letter each second it would take about one hundred years to read all the DNA in those forty-six chromosomes. We have about thirty thousand genes and more than 99 percent of these are exactly the same in each and every human being. It's the few that are different that create the differences among us and explain why one person will respond to a drug and another will not. Or why one person will have no side effects while the same drug in another person will cause major toxicity. But more about this later. What I hope you have gathered so far is that DNA is indeed the "code of life" and that our new understanding of the genome will open many previously closed doors.

IMPLICATIONS OF GENOMICS ON MEDICAL CARE

Still to come is to understand the exact sequence (those coded four letters A, T, C, and G) in each of the thirty thousand genes and to determine the function of each gene.

As this is done during the coming years, it will become possible to predict who might be more susceptible to a disease, such as atherosclerosis (clogging of the heart's blood vessels), diabetes, or perhaps colon cancer. Knowing that a person is at higher risk will allow the physician to recommend a preventive approach, such as diet and lifestyle changes, for each of these diseases—attention to cholesterol levels for the person at risk for atherosclerosis, weight control for the person predisposed to diabetes, and to an early start with screening colonoscopies for the person at risk of colon cancer. It will allow drug companies to create specific drugs to counter a disease while avoiding unwanted side effects and will allow the physician to choose the drug that will be known to work in a given patient and known not to cause any unwanted toxicities.

As we'll see as we move forward, genomics also is allowing scientists to better understand bacteria and viruses. For example, remember when the serious infection SARS started in Southeast Asia a few years ago and quickly spread to a number of distant cities such as Toronto, Canada? Microbiologists were able to quite quickly figure out the entire genome of that virus. That helped them understand how it would spread and infect—and possibly how it could be treated. Luckily, the SARS epidemic died out, but not before scientists discovered the nature of this particular "bug" faster than had ever been done before.

Genomics also has led to *gene expression profiling,* a new technique that we'll discuss later. But in a nutshell, gene expression profiling creates an opportunity to understand a tumor in much more detail. Scientists can determine if it is likely to spread or not (which aids in determining the long-term prognosis) and as a result recommend proper therapy. Profiling will also allow us to determine the risk of a disease, such as a heart attack *(acute myocardial infarction),* and genomic analysis will let us look at how a person is likely to respond to a drug, such as those used for seizures.

I suspect it will be some time before there will be much true gene therapy, that is, the insertion of a new gene to counteract for a deficit or abnormal gene. So in the meantime, medicine will focus on changing the environment rather than the genetics. If we know that a person won't respond to albuterol, then we can simply prescribe a different drug.

If we can identify a gene, then we can move on to identify what proteins or enzymes the gene produces and what that protein or enzyme actually does inside the cell. With that information we can then create a diagnostic test and from that either develop a preventive approach or we could modify the treatment. So in Anna's case it will one day be possible with a simple finger stick in the doctor's office to know that she will not respond to albuterol. In her case the doctor would prescribe a different drug.

Another result of identifying a gene and then its protein product is that we can now understand the basic defect in a disease and as a result create a specific drug. We can call this approach to medicine "targeted therapy." *Chronic myelocytic leukemia* (CML) is a good example. Two pieces from two chromosomes that have broken off rearrange themselves so that the piece from the first chromosome—containing part of a normal gene called BCR—attaches to the other chromosome next to a normal gene called ABL, creating a new gene and hence a new protein, each called BCR-ABL. The problem is that this is not a normal protein, and this new protein is what causes the disease we call chronic myelocytic leukemia.

The abnormal BCR-ABL protein allows this one cell to divide and divide and then divide again until eventually there are millions and then billions of these abnormal cells in the person's body. Until now, the approach to treating this disease has been to use fairly aggressive forms of cancer chemotherapy to kill off the dividing cells. But these drugs all have their own side effects, and they kill off other dividing cells as well. Knowing the underlying gene (BCR-ABL) and its protein product (BCR-ABL protein) and using some sophisticated techniques, such as nuclear magnetic resonance imaging and X-ray crystallography, researchers determined the site of the active protein—the part that causes something to happen, such as cell division. With this information in hand, scientists found a compound that would neatly insert itself into this active site, blocking the action of the protein. This compound, *Gleevec*, has had a major impact on those who suffer with chronic myelocytic leukemia.

Taking the drug blocks this active site and hence the disease seems to "disappear." Of course, because the underlying abnormal gene is still there, it will continue to produce the abnormal protein. But as long as the patient takes Gleevec, the abnormal protein's action is suppressed. This is one of the first examples of what is known as "targeted therapy," meaning that the drug is selected specifically because it blocks the action of this very specific abnormal protein.

In the past, if drugs were found to be effective and free of major side effects, then they could be used for whatever conditions seemed to respond. The difference here is in precisely knowing the activity of the BCR-ABL protein and what it does that is abnormal in the cell—and then learning what the active site is and how to specifically block it. (The Novartis Corporation actually had the drug Gleevec on its shelves. Developed for a different purpose years ago, it didn't work. But when scientists discovered the active site of the BCR-ABL protein, they were able to review a large drug database and determine that Gleevec might well be what was needed. And indeed it was.)

PHARMACOGENOMICS

All this is leading to *pharmacogenomics,* a new field that will create these targeted therapies. Watch the newspapers and magazines, and during the coming years you'll see quite a few drugs that have been created to respond to an understanding of how the protein actually works within the cell. The new science of genomics will also give us some other opportunities to advance medicine.[3]

We will be able to determine in advance whether a drug will work and whether it will work in a specific person. Likewise we'll be able to determine in advance whether a drug will cause side effects or toxicities in an individual person. This is the beginning of what some are terming "personalized medicine." Will a drug work? Let's return to Anna Blumenthal, her asthma, and albuterol.

Genomics Will Change the Approach to Drug Therapy

- Right Drug
- Right Patient—Improved Safety
- Right Time
- Increased Efficacy

Albuterol is commonly used in acute attacks of asthma to open the airways. Most people respond well within a short period of time. Some individuals will respond, but clearly not as well as the majority of folks. And then there is that small minority of people, like Anna, who get no response or even have a sense that the asthma has gotten worse. Until now we could only detect that small minority by trial and error, as happened with Anna.

Two o'clock in the morning when you're alone and scared is not the time to discover that you're in that small minority of people who won't respond. Why didn't Anna respond to the albuterol as nearly everyone else does? *Beta-adrenergic receptor,* a protein, is on the airways going into the lungs. Usually, when albuterol comes in contact with this receptor, the two bind together, and the result is that the smooth muscles surrounding the airways relax. This protein receptor is the product of its gene, which at codon number 27 (remember those three-letter codes for individual amino acids?) normally has the code for arginine. But sometimes one of those A, T, C, and G letters is substituted, which is just enough to change the code at number 27 from normally inserting the amino acid arginine into the protein at that point, to one of inserting the amino acid glycine into the protein.

If our beta-adrenergic receptor has a glycine at number 27 rather than arginine, there is little or no response to albuterol. But remember, we get half of our genes from Mom and half from Dad, so chances are that if one of our parents gave us the code for glycine, it's likely that the other parent still gave us the more common code for arginine. In this case, half of our receptors would be responsive—and half would not—when we come in contact with albuterol. As a result we would get some response, but a reduced response compared to normal. If we were to be like Anna and get the gene that codes for glycine from *both* Mom and Dad, then we would get no response at all to the albuterol. The good news is that this is now understood, and it is reasonable to predict that a simple blood test will be available in the not-too-distant future that will identify people like Anna who won't respond.

Here's another example. We all know that we should have our cholesterol checked and if it's high begin a program of appropriate diet and exercise to bring it down. That's not sufficient for some people and a type of drug called *statins* can be effective. The way to find out if you'll respond to a statin is to take it for a few months and then check to see how your cholesterol is doing. But statins are expensive, especially the newer ones that are under patent. You could literally spend hundreds, if not thousands, of dollars before finding out that a particular statin does not work for you.

The TV ads for statins briefly mention, "If you should develop muscle aches and pains tell your doctor" and comment, "A simple blood test will check for liver problems." The TV ads make these side effects sound trivial and it's true that they are rare, but when problems occur they are actually quite serious. If it happens to you, then suddenly it is not rare.

A gene that produces an enzyme (protein) is a critical part of our body's ability to control cholesterol. So far we know of at least two mutations to this gene that result in statins having a reduced effect. A person with one of these mutations who starts taking a statin will have a reduction of total cholesterol, LDL cholesterol (the "bad" cholesterol) and triglycerides, but it will be much less than the average person. Given the high cost of statins and the unlikely but real potential for toxicities, wouldn't it make sense to have a test done before starting a statin to make sure that you will respond and benefit from the drug? The result of such testing would mean safer and more effective therapy—this is the promise of genomics.

The understanding of the genome is creating a wealth of data on why some individuals respond differently to commonly used drugs. Following are a few examples to illustrate how genomics will lead to better and safer drug therapy in the future as physicians write out their prescriptions.

Some time in your life you've probably taken codeine, perhaps after having a tooth extracted. The dentist gave you a prescription, you took the codeine, and the pain got better. That's what usually happens, but there are a few people who start to have breathing difficulty. This side effect has long been known to occur, but why it occurred and in whom it would occur was unknown. The worst time to find out that the codeine is not going to work for you is when you also have an ache in your jaw from the extraction. But there has been no way to know in advance and, since it isn't common, physicians and dentists have not worried about it too much.

The cause relates to minor differences in the gene that codes for an enzyme located in the liver. This enzyme metabolizes or transforms codeine into morphine. Morphine is actually the active pain killer and is substantially more potent than codeine. But morphine is also well known to depress breathing if given in high doses. So if the codeine converts rapidly to morphine, then breathing difficulties can occur. We now know that some people have a slightly different gene for this enzyme, making their liver enzyme work faster and making them prone to this adverse event.

Here's another example related to the commonly used anticancer drug 5-fluorocytosine (5-FU). Someone in a distant city called one day to say that his father had colon cancer and that following surgery he had been given 5-FU to combat residual cancer. He was now in the local hospital intensive care unit because the standard dose of 5-FU that he had been given had acted as if it were a much larger dose and had caused severe ulcerations in his mouth and all along his intestinal tract. This in turn led to serious infections and he was critically ill.

The son asked if I could talk to the oncologist just to be sure that he was getting the best possible care. I happen to know the oncologist is very competent. It turned out that he was indeed getting excellent care and that the oncologist was deeply distressed that the 5-FU had had this unexpected and certainly unwanted side effect. What had happened?

5-FU is usually given by mouth or by vein and works to block cell division, a useful benefit in patients where the cancer cells are rapidly dividing. But we have other dividing cells in the body, including the cells that line our mouth and intestines. As a result, high doses of 5-FU over a prolonged period can cause painful mouth ulcers, diarrhea, and other changes to the intestines, along with causing hair loss and reduction in the production of red blood cells, white blood cells, and platelets. Physicians are therefore very careful to give enough, but not too much, 5-FU.

An enzyme in the liver[4] breaks down 5-FU into inactive compounds that are then excreted by the body. In some rare individuals there can be a fatal or near-fatal reaction to customary doses. When this occurs it is shocking, especially since it cannot be predicted.

If either Mom or Dad pass on a gene encoded for this liver enzyme in an altered state, then we would only have one-half of the total amount of the enzyme working normally. The gene from say, Mom, would make an inactive enzyme whereas the one from Dad would be active. Half as much normal enzyme is not quite enough, and a patient receiving a normal dose of 5-FU would have some increase in toxicity. This is the situation in about 1 percent of the population.

On the other hand—and this is uncommon—if *both* Mom and Dad passed on the gene for the inactive enzyme, which is what happens in about 0.001 percent of the population, then the 5-FU would remain in the bloodstream at a high level for a long time with devastating results. Fortunately this is a very rare occurrence, but that's no consolation to the person who is affected, or to his or her loved ones after the fact. This enzyme has now been characterized and the gene for its production has been identified and cloned. It is now possible to determine, therefore, in advance of giving 5-FU, whether an individual has the abnormal gene and is consequently at risk.

Unfortunately, this test is not yet widely available and it is expensive. Presumably this will change with time as more physicians request it and more patients demand to be tested first. The chance of being in the high-risk group (0.001 percent) is obviously small, but in the case of my acquaintance, his father died of these side effects. He knows that he will certainly be tested should he ever need 5-FU.

Another set of genes—for a set of enzymes (cytochrome P-450) in the liver—determines how the body will metabolize or break down drugs such as those in the class called *selective serotonin inhibitors* (SSRIs). These drugs include common antidepressants like Prozac and Zoloft. For most individuals the usual dose is just fine, but for others a difference in their cytochrome P-450 activity means that they can actually be taking a dose of Prozac or Zoloft that's much too high for them and hence they'll have side effects. Actually, this liver enzyme has two types and they are key to how our body breaks down (metabolizes) many drugs.

Those who have the genome that results in an excessive amount of this enzyme are *ultrarapid metabolizers*. Most of us are in the categories known as "extensive" or "intermediate" metabolizers, meaning we have about the average amount of this enzyme present in our liver. Others who have little or even a total absence of this enzyme are known as "poor" metabolizers. It's probably obvious that those who are poor metabolizers will have higher concentrations of some drugs in their bloodstream for too long, leading to toxicities.

On the other side of the coin, for the ultrarapid metabolizers, some drugs are hard to keep in a high concentration in the bloodstream. For example, the antibiotics used to treat the bacterium (*Heliobacter pylori* or *H. pylori* for short) that causes stomach ulcers need to be in high concentration. So people with lower levels of this cytochrome P-450 enzyme will actually respond better to these antibiotics. And remember our discussion about codeine? Those who too rapidly convert it to morphine can have breathing problems, but at the other end of the spectrum, those who convert it slowly will get less pain relief.

Similar to 5-FU, another anticancer drug can have severe adverse effects in a small minority of individuals. *6-mercaptopurine* (6-MP) is commonly used to treat children with acute leukemia. Indeed it is one of the mainstays in the drug armamentarium for that disease. A very small number of these children develop exceptionally severe side effects. It's as though the drug was given in a much higher dose than actually was given. The reason is that the drug remains for much too long in the bloodstreams of children who fall into the category of poor metabolizers.

The result is that the 6-MP will damage the bone marrow so that red blood cells, white blood cells, and platelets are not produced as they should be; it may also damage the intestinal tract and the mouth as occurred in the gentleman who was taking 5-FU. These children become exceptionally ill and sometimes die of this apparent "overdose." Until recently there was just no way to know who would have this type of response until it actually happened. Now with the ability to test in advance for the level of cytochrome P-450 the oncologist will know to give this child a greatly reduced dose of the 6-MP.

There is now a fairly simple test for the cytochrome P-450 enzymes. It's a quick and direct test and should reduce the chance for adverse effects from antidepressants, give a better idea of the proper dose in treating *H. pylori* infection, properly reduce the dose for the child with leukemia taking 6-MP, and identify those who will react adversely or not adequately to codeine.

Today a drug company enlists patients with an illness or a condition, such as high cholesterol, to be studied with an investigational drug, such as a statin. But wouldn't it be useful to know in advance how that patient might be expected to respond? Based on predictive metabolism or excretion, researchers could determine whether the drug is likely to have the desired effect in that patient, or possibly have an unwanted side effect. It would mean many fewer patients needed to complete a clinical trial, substantially reducing the cost and time to get a new drug on the market. With genomics, understanding how a drug works in the body may well make it possible to do just that.

This approach could eliminate potential subjects who likely will not respond to a drug and potentially assure that the new drug is only tested in those individuals where it's likely to have a good effect and little or no toxicity. This differs significantly from clinical trials today. It would in effect say that a drug is being designed for a specific purpose to affect a specific target and that it will only be used among patients who have that target (protein or enzyme) in their bodies. Drug trials could be done with fewer individuals and in less time.

Pharmacogenomics

■ Using Genomic Information
  — Drug companies can create drugs with
    • Specificity
    • Safety
  — Physicians can select prescription based upon
    • Individual genomic testing
      – Drug that is active in *that* person
      – Drug that is safe in *that* person

It should become evident sooner whether the drug is effective for the disease in question and side effects should be much less common. The drug company, in setting up the clinical trial, would include genomic tests to determine the presence of the target and also a test to determine how the drug might be metabolized.

NUTRAGENOMICS

Let's turn now from pharmacogenomics to nutragenomics. Our genes also affect how we respond to the various foods we eat, just as they affect how we respond to the drugs we take. We all seem to know that person who can eat anything and never gain weight. Or the person who eats all the things that we've learned not to eat—the high cholesterol foods like a hamburger and fries—and yet has no problem with coronary artery disease or gout. The answer would seem to be in our genes. Human details aren't worked out yet. But in mice, those lacking the gene SCD-1 are apparently genetically safe and can eat all the fatty foods they want without developing obesity or diabetes.

People have a set of genes called apoEs that create one of three proteins (also known as apoEs) important in the metabolism of cholesterol. The specific version of the three different types of apoE genes you carry makes a big difference in how you respond to the foods that you eat. More than one-half of the population has apoE3, the "normal" gene that produces the "normal" protein. ApoE4, less common, affecting about 20 to 40 percent of the population, has a single codon difference at #158, which directs the amino acid cysteine instead of arginine in the protein.

Such an apparently minimal difference creates a big difference in how a person metabolizes cholesterol; it creates a two-sided sword. Those who carry this gene tend to have higher cholesterol levels and are at greater risk for coronary artery disease and heart attack. But on the positive side, people who carry this gene variant can significantly reduce that risk by eating a healthy, low-fat, low-cholesterol diet. A high-fat, high-cholesterol diet will shoot up their bad cholesterol (LDL cholesterol) but a healthy diet will push the LDL cholesterol level way down. Even though this person has the adverse gene for coronary artery disease, they can significantly reduce their risk with a healthy diet.[5]

Individuals with the apoE3 or the other variant apoE2 have less risk from a high-fat diet, but conversely it's harder for them to drive down their cholesterol levels through a healthy diet. Maybe understanding these and other genetic patterns will suggest who might do better with the Ornish low-fat diet or the Atkins low-carbohydrate diet.

GENOMICS AND PREDICTION OF LATER DISEASE DEVELOPMENT

Genetic tests that can predict the potential development of a disease later in life are rapidly being developed. What options are available now? How useful are they? Here are some answers.

Let's use breast and ovarian cancer as examples. Of all women who develop breast cancer, about 2 to 3 percent have inherited either of two mutated genes known as BCRA-1 (breast cancer susceptibility gene 1) or BCRA-2. Both of these genes substantially increase a woman's risk of developing breast or ovarian cancer or both. Those with either gene have a 60 to 85 percent lifetime risk of breast cancer, and a 15 to 60 percent lifetime risk of ovarian cancer.

This is much higher than in the general population of women for whom the lifetime risk is about 9 percent for breast cancer and less than 1 percent for ovarian cancer. When women with either of these two mutated genes develop these cancers they tend to occur earlier in life and also tend to spread more aggressively. These genes are also more prevalent in Ashkenazi Jews— those with a central or eastern European ancestry.

Who should be tested to see if they carry the BCRA-1 or BCRA-2 genes?

And what should a woman do if she's found to be positive for one of these genes? At this time, it would seem reasonable for a woman with a strong history of breast cancer in her family (two or more of mother, sister, aunt, etc.) or any history of ovarian cancer in the family to be tested. Those who test positive for BCRA-1 or BCRA-2 should then plan to be checked regularly for breast cancer so it can be detected and treated at the earliest stages. Another option is prophylactic mastectomies.

For those opting for the mammography route, this should be started at about age thirty, compared to the usual recommendation for most women to start screening mammography at age forty. Another approach to mammography is to use magnetic resonance imaging (MRI). This takes longer and is much more costly than routine mammography, so MRI would normally not be used for screening purposes (see the chapter on imaging). But it is more sensitive, and so in these women it might be a wise choice given their increased risk. A routine mammogram can probably pick up about 70 percent of small cancers, whereas MRI may be sensitive enough to detect 95 percent.

Unfortunately, everything good seems to come with a downside. In this case the high sensitivity of the MRI also picks up masses that are not cancerous (we call this having a *lower specificity* than do regular mammograms). The result is that someone may end up with a biopsy that proves to be negative. The question for an individual woman thinking about having an MRI performed for screening is whether she's prepared to accept the possibility that there will be a false positive report requiring a biopsy that later will prove to be negative. Some would say that's a small hurdle for those who are at higher risk and others would say it's an unnecessary added burden and stress.

No good screening test exists for ovarian cancer. Indeed, ovarian cancer is usually detected only after it has spread to other locations. For this reason, many specialists would recommend that a BCRA-1 or a BCRA-2 test-positive woman have her ovaries surgically removed after she has completed childbearing. A recent study of 1,828 BRCA-1 or BRCA-2 positive women showed an 80 percent reduction in occurrence of ovarian cancer after *oophorectomy* (ovary and fallopian tube removal).[6]

This, of course, needs to be weighed against the risk of surgery and the symptoms of early menopause that the removal will cause. A possible alternative is to have annual ultrasound exams. Today's ultrasound equipment theoretically should be able to pick up ovarian cancer if done routinely, especially with a vaginal probe. But studies to date have not demonstrated that this technique picks up these tumors before they've spread to distant locations.

The important lesson is that a small subset of women is at much higher risk of breast and ovarian cancer than the general population. Since there's actually something that can be done either to prevent these tumors from ever occurring (prophylactic surgery) or to find them when they're tiny (screening techniques), it follows that the genetic test is useful.

Researchers are rapidly bearing in on the genetic basis of diabetes. Diabetes is not caused solely by our genetic background, but genetics has a powerful influence on whether environmental factors will be able to cause it. Much of this type of work is based on looking for *single nucleotide polymorphisms* (SNPs). There are about three billion base pairs in our DNA and about one out of each one thousand varies between any two individuals. This means that there are about three million variations between any two individuals.

Researchers are trying to learn which ones produce disease and which ones predict disease. With the advanced technologies available today it is possible to do assays on a person's DNA that can look at five hundred thousand SNPs at once, do it all in about six hours, and at a cost of only about one cent per SNP.

Within the next ten years or so, look for the ability for each of us to have our entire genome analyzed for about one thousand dollars. Then all of this information will be available for prediction and prevention.

GENOMICS AND PREDICTING DISEASE PROGRESSION

Before discussing the specifics, it will help to understand a powerful new laboratory tool that makes genomics medically useful. The technique uses microarray technologies. Here's basically how it works.

Recall that when a gene in the DNA turns on, it makes mRNA, which goes into the cell's "factory" to make a protein. For our microarray testing, a scientist puts a tiny drop of DNA from a single gene on a glass slide and then covers it with the mRNA of a sample, let's say, from a cancer biopsy. If the mRNA from the tumor sample is complementary to the DNA originally placed on the slide, then the two compounds will interact. If there's a lot of this mRNA in the sample, then there will be a lot of interaction, whereas if there's relatively little mRNA, then there will be minimal interaction.

In the case of a lot of mRNA, this would represent that gene being "turned on" and being "overexpressed." On the other hand, if there's relatively little mRNA coming from the tumor sample, then that gene is "turned off" and is being "underexpressed." Think of it simply as a way of determining if a gene is active—or not—at a given time in a given tissue.

In the previous example, we looked at just one gene. The microarray technology allows for literally thousands of genes or gene fragments to be analyzed simultaneously—all on one tiny glass slide—to determine whether they are turned on or turned off. Following are a few examples of what gene expression through microarray technology can yield.

First, it holds promise that patients with breast cancer can be better identified as to who needs or does not need chemotherapy after surgery and radiation therapy. Obviously this is a critical issue for the patient and her physician, who face a major decision. Basically the tumor describes its own "molecular signature" with the gene expression profiling. One signature represents a bad prognosis (i.e., about 60% have a recurrence) and hence a patient who should get aggressive chemotherapy. Another signature represents a good prognosis and thus a woman who may not need chemotherapy at all.

In patients with early stage lung cancer, there are data that when tested for their tumor's molecular/genomic signatures, patients can be placed into two very disparate groups of good versus bad prognosis based on these genomic assays; that is, one group has a survival rate after surgery of nearly 90% whereas the others nearly all die within four to five years.

These observations are still investigational, but there is clear hope that this will become mainstream in just a few years and benefit each woman who develops breast cancer or each man or woman who develops lung cancer.[7]

For our second example, consider the virtual epidemic of reflux esophagitis. This refers to acid from the stomach flowing up into the esophagus where it damages the cell lining and can cause the pain we call heartburn. Over time, some people with reflux esophagitis will develop a change in the cells in the lower esophagus that has the potential to progress to cancer. Pathologists call this "Barrett's esophagus," and it, too, is increasing in recent years.

No one knows all the reasons, but we do know that a small percentage of those with acid reflux will progress to the changes seen on biopsy that are characteristic of Barrett's, and then in turn some of these individuals will develop esophageal cancer. But we do not know who will progress to Barrett's or who will progress to overt cancer. Soon, with the use of gene expression profiling using microarray technology, it may be possible to determine which person with Barrett's is at increased risk of progressing to cancer and which patient is not.

GENOMICS TO IMPROVE DIAGNOSIS
AND PROGNOSTICATION

Let's use examples of leukemia, colon cancer, and lymphoma to see how genomics will play a critical role in the future in diagnosing and predicting the course of these diseases.

It's sometimes difficult for the pathologist or hematologist to differentiate acute myelocytic leukemia from acute lymphocytic leukemia. The differentiation is critical because we use different drugs for these two types of acute leukemia. Using the new microarray technologies, it is now becoming possible to determine which genes are over- or underexpressed in each patient. The genomic assay technology shows quite different expression patterns between acute myelocytic leukemia and acute lymphocytic leukemia. In all likelihood this technique shortly will be available as a mainstream diagnostic aid for acute leukemia, assuring that each patient gets the correct therapy from the start. In addition, genomic analyses can place patients into prognostic categories as to the likelihood of responding to standard treatments.[8]

When individuals have a colon cancer removed by surgery, frequently the cancer has spread somewhat across the layers of the intestine. It's known that this type of spread, although apparently only in the bowel wall itself, may in some patients be a harbinger of microscopic disease elsewhere, such as in the liver. In other words, the tumor may have already spread even though we can't detect it at this time. As a result, all such patients receive a recommendation for *adjuvant chemotherapy*. We use the term *adjuvant* to mean that we can't prove that microscopic disease is present but it is reasonably likely, and therefore it's best to undergo the chemotherapy before the disease starts to grow. The best time to try to eradicate cancer is when there are only a few cells, not when the few have grown into multiple large masses.

The problem is that not all patients need this adjuvant therapy. But there has been no way to differentiate who does and who does not. With microarray technologies it may soon be possible to identify which patient has a tumor that is likely to have spread and therefore needs the chemotherapy. The patient with a cancer that in all likelihood has not spread can be spared the side effects of unnecessary drug treatment. This will be a true advance in medicine.

Think about genomics and medicine this way: only the correct drug will be selected for an individual patient; the drug will be given at the correct time relative to the patient's own needs, resulting in increased effectiveness and much-improved safety with fewer side effects. Here's another example of how genomics can help determine the appropriate treatment. Lymphomas are cancers that arise in the lymph nodes. The most widely known among them is Hodgkin's disease, but the most common form in adults is *diffuse large B-cell lymphoma*. The name is derived from its appearance under the microscope— the tumor is diffusely infiltrating a lymph node, the cells are relatively large compared to other lymphocytes, and they are of B-cell origin. (There are two types of lymphocytes, B- and T-cell.)

About 35 to 40 percent of patients with diffuse large B-cell lymphoma can be cured with a combination of drugs. Other patients with tumors that appear identical respond less positively when given the exact same drugs and usually die after a few years. It's been impossible to know in advance which patients will do well and which will not. Researchers suspect that multiple diseases masquerade with a similar anatomic appearance under the microscope.

If a patient could be classified at the time of diagnosis as one who will not respond well to standard chemotherapy, then more aggressive therapy—possibly newer investigational drugs or a marrow or stem cell transplant—could be considered. In short, different therapeutic approaches could be entertained from the start, rather than after months of unsuccessful chemotherapy has taken its toll with all of its side effects and toxicities.

In recent years microarray technology has begun to make a prognostic differentiation. Investigators at the National Cancer Institute retrieved stored biopsy samples from patients who had been treated some years ago. They then did microarray gene expression profiling and found that they could divide patients into subgroups that closely related to how long the patients survived after treatment.[9] So it should be possible for a person with newly diagnosed lymphoma to find out how he or she will likely respond to standard therapy or whether it would be appropriate to receive more aggressive therapy. This technique of gene expression profiling will certainly be improved in the coming years and will undoubtedly become mainstream in the near future.

MOLECULAR DIAGNOSTICS

Molecular diagnostics will revolutionize medicine as a result of the genomic era. We've already talked about how DNA microarrays can be used in differentiating whether an individual person who has developed Barrett's changes of their esophagus as a result of gastric acid reflux likely will or will not develop cancer. And we've seen how DNA microarrays in diffuse large B-cell lymphomas will differentiate those who are likely to respond to chemotherapy from those who are not as likely to respond, despite the fact that their tumors look identical under the microscope.

In both cases this involved looking at literally thousands of genes or gene fragments to find patterns and to use these patterns or "molecular signatures" to differentiate. At this time we really don't know what each gene does or even which gene is most important in encouraging Barrett's to develop into cancer or one lymphoma to respond compared to another. The patterns do correlate with the underlying nature of the disease—how the disease will or will not spread and how it may or may not respond to therapy.

We've also discussed how gene analysis—or analysis of the protein produced by a gene—can determine who will have a side effect from a drug, who will have a positive or not-so-positive response to a drug, and who will respond to the new targeted drugs. For example, Herceptin (the brand name for the chemical *trastuzumab*) helps some patients with breast cancer. It inhibits a specific growth-related protein that's found only in some patients with breast cancer. This growth factor, HER-2/neu, is overexpressed in some but not all patients with breast cancer. So only those with the overexpression would respond to Herceptin.

We've also talked about the drug Gleevec, used for patients with chronic myelocytic leukemia because they have that specific abnormal gene called BCR-ABL, which in turn makes the abnormal BCR-ABL protein that Gleevec inhibits. Here, too, we would only want to use it for patients with that specific genetic change and hence that specific abnormal protein.

DESIGNER VACCINES

The term *designer vaccine* means that it is made especially for a given person. Following is an example of such a vaccine that is under development. Chronic lymphocytic leukemia (CLL) usually is an indolent (slowly progressive) tumor. Multiple drugs are used to treat it, but it is still incurable. So scientists are trying to find a way to eliminate the remaining leukemic cells. CLL—probably like all cancers—begins with one cell having the needed genomic change(s) that the cell requires to divide forever, without the normal regulatory checks and balances. We call this a *clone* of cells that originated from a single cell.

The question is how to eliminate all the cells of that clone and leave normal cells alone. Surgery may work for a solid tumor that has not spread. Radiation might do the same. Chemotherapy will destroy dividing cells, but often we can't give enough drugs because the drugs will also destroy too many normal dividing cells. So here is a new approach. Since CLL arises from a lymphocyte and since lymphocytes make an antibody, take the leukemic cell and extract the segment of the antibody that is "variable," that is, find the specific antibody that the leukemia cells—and only that clone of cells—makes. Take the gene out of the cell that makes this variable part of the antibody. Now use this DNA fragment as a vaccine. Inject it back into the patient with the idea that it will now immunize the patient to produce cells that will attack and destroy the CLL cells.

Will it work? I don't know. But this is a concept developed at the NIH National Institute of Aging and is being tested now on animals. In a few years, we will learn the answer. I use it as an example of the types of approaches that can be taken to create personal vaccines.

SOCIAL AND ETHICAL ISSUES OF THE GENOMIC ERA

It won't be too many years before it will be possible to have our own genome sequenced, probably at a fairly reasonable price. With this information, we can be told about our risk for various diseases, our likelihood to respond to various drugs, and so on. But will we want to have this information? If an insurer were to find that we were at high risk of heart disease, would they then cancel our life insurance policy or limit our health insurance policy? What about employers? Will they insist on seeing the results of our genomic analysis and make hiring or job classification decisions based on that information?

What if you were to develop diffuse large B-cell lymphoma and a genomic analysis showed that you were in a "poor" prognostic group? It probably would be good for you to get into a clinical trial at a major cancer center, but perhaps your insurer would say that it doesn't want to pay for any therapy since it probably won't work. These are difficult questions that are even more difficult to answer. Hopefully our social and ethical deliberations and decisions will move along at a rate somewhat close to the rapid rate at which genomics is advancing.

And of course, it raises the issue of health care costs. Genomic analysis will cost money. Will it be worth it? I would argue that if you are the person who has an alternative to albuterol in the middle of the night or if you are the patient who, after genomic testing, is not given a standard dose of 5-FU or 6-MP because you would metabolize it in a way that could kill you, then you will find the cost worthwhile. But if you are in the vast majority of people who respond to albuterol or have a normal reaction to 5-FU or 6-MP, then from your perspective the extra testing is an added expense that wasn't needed. The answers to these difficult issues are not clear or easy, but it is clear that the start of the genomic medicine era is revolutionizing medicine.

MEGATRENDS RELATED TO GENOMICS

With the dawning of the genomic era, expect your doctor to have much improved capabilities to diagnose disease, to predict your future health based on your personal genome, and to be able to estimate or prognosticate what your disease will do if left alone or if treated with one approach versus another.

THE MEGATRENDS

- ■ "Personalized Medicine" Will Arrive
- ■ Much Improved Diagnosis including Molecular Diagnosis
- ■ Predict Future Onset of Disease
- ■ Predict Disease Progression
- ■ Gene Therapy Will Begin
- ■ Predict Responses to Drugs
- ■ Create Targeted Drugs
- ■ Drugs Will Become More Effective, More Specific, Safer and Have Fewer Side Effects

Drug therapy will become more effective, more specific, safer, and have fewer side effects. Many drugs will be created with a specific target based on the knowledge gained from genomic analyses and an understanding of the protein that a specific gene creates. Vaccines will be designed for the individual patient to treat some types of cancer and vaccines will be created to treat other diseases like multiple sclerosis, diabetes, rheumatoid arthritis, and possibly even atherosclerosis, drug addiction, and Alzheimer's. And finally, we will see the beginning of actual gene therapy—replacing a gene that causes disease with the proper gene to return the person to a state of health. All this will occur in the not-too-distant future. These are truly transformational changes that will occur in medical practice, ones that will disrupt the current "normal" approach to health care and offer the opportunity for a much more personalized form of care.

WHAT YOU SHOULD KNOW ABOUT GENOMICS

You should understand how DNA works and how it does indeed represent "the code of life." You should have a sense of how the genomic era will predict disease in a specific individual, such as identifying a risk of heart attack or of colon cancer at an early age. You should then understand how that genomic information can be used to prevent the disease, for example, by prescribing a low-fat diet to reduce the chance of a heart attack. Or how that knowledge will allow for prescribing a specific therapy for a disease or problem—for example, the use of Herceptin in selected patients with breast cancer based on the genomic profile of their tumor.

Knowledge of genes and their functions will lead to using gene therapy to replace defective genes. Understanding cellular receptors will determine what drug an individual should or should not take. Developing designer vaccines will address the special needs of patients, such as those with cancer. Genomics will help diagnose the presence of various diseases or, in the case of cancer, their likelihood of spreading (metastasizing) or responding to standard therapies. These are just some of the advances in medicine that will come from the knowledge gained in the coming years from genomics.

What about gene therapy? Will we be able to treat a disease caused by a genetic mutation with a new gene? The time will come when this will be possible; how soon is not clear. It sounds easy, but in practice it may be a lot more complicated than previously thought—and risky.

My grandfather spent most of his career diagnosing disease so that he could explain to the patient and family what was happening and what likely would happen as a result of the disease—since he could do little to treat it.

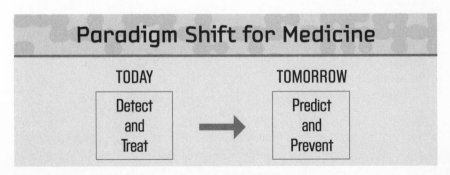

During most of my career in the late twentieth century, medicine was all about detecting a disease so that it could be treated with increasingly sophisticated approaches. In the genomic era, the physician may spend the bulk of his or her time predicting that a disease will occur and then working with the patient on a preventive regimen. Maybe the physician will prescribe a medication, lifestyle changes, a complementary medicine approach, or a dietary supplement. This will be a truly fundamental change in the practice of medicine. And it will be individualized for each of us—*personalized medicine*.

WHAT YOU CAN DO

Armed with this new information, you as a patient or potential patient should first keep your eyes open for articles in the newspapers or in magazines about new advances based on genomics. Second, be sure to query your physician about how genomic analyses might benefit you if you develop a disease, need a new drug, or just want to understand your risk for the future. It's always a good idea to come to your physician with your questions thought out and the subject as well versed in your mind as possible. Use the Internet to collect information, but only use highly trustworthy sources, such as the National Institutes of Health Web site.[10]

But remember that this is a fast-developing and changing field so your physician may not be as up-to-date as you are on specific information. Make it a sharing opportunity, but also remember that your physician will take that information and integrate it into everything else he or she knows about you and your illness, along with all of the knowledge and experience that has gone before. In short, don't try to be your own physician, but do be prepared. The end result will be much better for you.

CHAPTER 2

Stem Cells and Regenerative Medicine—The Promise of the Future

Peter Morningstar, forty-one, the director of physical therapy at a suburban rehabilitation center, had been feeling tired and then noticed red spots on his legs. Reluctantly, he visited his doctor and learned that he had acute myelocytic leukemia, which is fatal if not treated and then fatal, eventually, because the disease comes back. Peter underwent three rounds of intensive chemotherapy. His hair fell out, his mouth hurt, and he had high fevers. He needed powerful intravenous antibiotics, and he required platelet and blood transfusions.

After five weeks, Peter received some good news: the leukemia cells were gone, and he was in what is called a *complete remission*. But how to prevent the disease from returning? He needed even more aggressive chemotherapy to kill off any remaining leukemia cells. The problem was, such high doses would kill all the cells in his bone marrow—including the stem cells that were responsible for making his red and white blood cells and his platelets. Without those blood cells, he would die.

Peter's doctor recommended he undergo a stem cell transplant. His sister had already had her cells tissue typed; their immune systems matched closely, and she could be the donor. He agreed, and the transplant was scheduled. A remarkable machine removed his sister's blood-forming stem cells by taking just those cells from her blood and putting everything else back into her veins. Meanwhile, Peter underwent more aggressive chemotherapy, in hopes of killing off the remaining leukemia cells hiding in his body.

When the drugs were out of his body, his sister's stem cells were injected into his vein. They seemed to know just where in his body to go, and within a few weeks, his bone marrow was making new blood cells again, but this time they were the progeny of his sister's stem cells rather than his own. The chemotherapy had totally destroyed his stem cells. Only time will tell, but hopefully, Peter is cured.

THE RESEARCH REVOLUTION AND REGENERATIVE MEDICINE

In this chapter I will review some of the basic science of stem cells and their potential to radically alter people's ability to heal. Stem cell therapy promises to be one of those true scientific breakthroughs that will impact future health care. Stem cell therapy will bring us closer to the goal of personalized medicine, just as genomics is doing. My intent is to clarify issues so that the adult versus embryonic stem cell debate can be rational and meaningful. I will, as suggested by Peter's story, describe how adult stem cells are already being used for treating some cancers and are being studied experimentally in the treatment of heart attack victims and certain tissue repairs.

Unlike the technologies of imaging and other devices or even genomics, the stem cell megatrend is further into the future—projections need to be five, ten, even twenty-five and more years out—because this is truly an emerging science. The course of a disease will change once we have the technology to insert stem cells into the human body to actually create a tissue. The generalized hope is that stem cells will provide a new approach to curative therapy of many diseases and less toxic therapy for many others. Organs and tissues that are damaged or diseased will be repaired or even replaced.

Today we insert artificial knees made of metal; tomorrow new cartilage cells will replace those destroyed by osteoarthritis or by weekend warrior injuries.

Today we are excited that new insulin pumps make the care of diabetes much easier; tomorrow replacement cells will make insulin for those in the pancreas that were lost. Today we can do a lot for individuals who have a heart attack—drugs, stents, surgery; tomorrow we may be able to heal the damaged muscle with stem cells. Today drugs can assist those with Parkinson's disease; tomorrow perhaps their symptoms will be gone after the insertion of new brain cells to replace those that are no longer functioning.

Today an orthopedist puts metal rods into a traumatized leg; tomorrow he or she will insert a total bone substitute that will regenerate the muscles and nerves around it. Sometimes tissue will be "grown" over a scaffold that creates the shape needed and then dissolves away after the new tissue is complete. This is the concept of regenerative medicine. To a large degree it is still far over the horizon, but science is moving fast and some of these techniques will become commonplace soon. Indeed, some already are, as Peter's story illustrates.

Human development is a complex process. How does a fertilized ovum ultimately become a person? How do these initially undifferentiated stem cells slowly become first committed to a certain type of tissue and then actually go on to form it? Genes must turn on and off, and we need to learn about them. Knowing how these mechanisms work will help us understand when the process sometimes goes wrong and a child is born with congenital heart disease, Down syndrome, or missing both arms.

If we know what goes wrong, maybe we can find ways to prevent it from occurring in the future. Or maybe even correct it afterward. Similarly, cancer starts with a stem cell that has become abnormal. What is that abnormality, and why did it occur? We know that for most cancers, genetic and environmental factors cause cells to change and become malignant, but what exactly are these changes, and how did they come about? Understanding how stem cells mature and progress to normal tissues or cancerous cells will give scientists a real boost in understanding and developing preventive and treatment approaches.

Stem cells one day may be useful for testing new drugs. If a steady supply of stem cells could in turn produce a steady supply of tissue cells, then a new drug could be tested on living cell cultures before being tested in humans.

This might allow for a consistent approach to learning how a drug interacts with a particular cell type. For example, one could develop an unending supply of exactly the same heart muscle cells. These could be used to test the effectiveness and the toxicities of new drugs for improving heart failure. Since the drugs would be used on heart muscle cells that are all the same, the results from drug to drug could be compared, speeding the process of learning the needed dose before ever moving on to animal studies or human trials.

These are the potentials that stem cells hold and this is the promise of regenerative medicine. From what we know today these are realistic potentials and realistic promises. But we should not lose balance in our enthusiasm for what is still in the future. It may be that after rigorous testing in the laboratories, what appears on the drawing boards to be an inevitable triumph of science will ultimately not match our expectations.

Peter's struggle (and the countless others like it) gives us some indication of and motivation for the benefits of stem cell research. Though Peter is back at work as an active health care practitioner in his rehabilitation center, his road was difficult, to say the least, and only time will tell if he is cured. As a society, we need to agree on what we will tolerate in order to make the research advance. To do so yourself with a balanced opinion we will continue with a review of what stem cells are, how they are obtained and worked with, and then what can be done with adult stem cells, embryonic stem cells, and possibly nuclear transfer stem cells. By the conclusion of this chapter, you will be in a better position to make your own informed decision as to the best course of national action regarding embryonic stem cells.

WHAT ARE STEM CELLS?

Most tissues or organs have a small number of cells—among their trillions of cells—that can each self-replicate or self-renew. Each time they divide, they can produce either two new stem cells or one stem cell and one cell destined to become the cell of that organ or tissue. These stem cells are the ones that actually create an organ or tissue during our fetal development, and the ones remaining in adult life are present to help regenerate or heal that specific tissue.

The concept of blood stem cells was first proposed around 1960. It was some years before their presence could be confirmed in mouse bone marrow, requiring the development of new technologies to identify and to select or isolate the stem cells from the larger pool of blood cells. So stem cells are relatively new in our understanding, but new information is coming at an increasingly rapid pace. For example, the same methods used to obtain stem cells from the blood or bone marrow were used to isolate stem cells from the brains of mice. These stem cells, able to self-renew, gave rise to all three types of brain (neural) cells. Further fascinating experiments showed that if these cells were injected into specific areas of the mouse brain, they would "take up residence" in that location, divide and develop into brain cells of that area's type, and then they would continue to replicate for the life of the mouse.

We know that human adult stem cells can be found in the bone marrow and blood and used as the story of Peter illustrates. More types of adult human stem cells have been discovered. We have learned that stem cells from some organs, like the bone marrow, can apparently become stem cells for many other organs, including the liver and heart. In 1998, human embryonic stem cells were isolated for the first time. Now the possibility exists for any of the body's more than two hundred cell types to be generated in the laboratory, presumably in an endless supply.

It has always been assumed that adult stem cells were only capable of producing "daughter" cells that would be of their own cell, organ, or tissue type—

that is, bone marrow stem cells make blood cells and liver stem cells make liver cells, and so forth. Now we are learning that some adult stem cells can become some other cell types—*pluripotent.* But embryonic stem cells can become any type of cell—*totipotent*—and that is why they hold such great promise.

The study of the miraculous abilities of embryonic and adult stem cells to regenerate the diseased organs of the body is just beginning, and many answers are still years away. It is my belief that stem cells do indeed promise to be one of the most significant advances ever made in the treatment of disease. But unlike some of the other revolutions discussed in other chapters, this one is still in its infancy. It will be many years before we will see cures of Parkinson's, diabetes, or heart disease. Yet stem cells are already having a beneficial effect.

Let me give you an example illustrating the potential of adult stem cells, which are without ethical controversy. In your imagination, accidentally cut off your middle finger. Discard the finger. You know you will never again have a usable middle finger of your own flesh and blood in that space. Now imagine cutting off a piece of your liver. Discard it too. Wait eight weeks. You will have your liver back again, completely restored. The liver is regenerated because stem cells found in the adult body are at work.

Certain tissue types seem to have them, and others do not, or at least, they cannot cause a tissue or organ to regrow. But bone marrow can regenerate itself if you bleed a large amount, and your liver can regrow to normal size if a section is surgically removed. In other cases, such as after a heart attack that damages heart muscle cells, some stem cells are present but are either not in sufficient numbers or cannot be adequately mobilized to repair the damaged heart muscle. Scientists are working to discover ways to activate inactive adult stem cells in other parts of the body, to regenerate healthy cells where needed.

As for that finger that was accidentally cut off—well, the cells in your hand do carry all of the genes that were present when your hand was developed as a fetus. Perhaps one day, we will learn how to stimulate cells to reform that finger. It is not beyond the realm of possibility.

Stem Cells: Where do they come from, and what do they do? The key characteristics of stem cells are that they can replicate themselves and they can become mature cells that make up the body. Embryonic stem cells can become any of the body's approximately two hundred types of cells (liver, lung, brain), and they have the capacity to divide or replicate indefinitely. Adult stem cells, as the name implies, can be found in the bodies of adults (or newborns and children). They also can self-replicate, but when placed in tissue culture, they have not replicated indefinitely as embryonic stem cells do.

When a fertilized egg begins the process of division, one cell becomes two, two become four, four become eight, and so forth. By the third to fifth day, there are many cells and they have divided into two sections. One section is called the *inner cell mass* of the blastocyst, which has about thirty to forty cells and is about the size of the period at the end of this sentence. These cells are the embryonic stem cells.

Each has the ability to become any cell or tissue of the body. Somehow, in the correct setting, which creates certain needed "signals," the individual cells of the inner cell mass will not only divide again and again, but will begin to differentiate—become more and more like the ultimate cell of the tissue or organ that they are destined to become. In effect but oversimplified, one cell's progeny will become the liver, one the heart, one the brain, and so on. This happens even though each cell contains the entire DNA complement. Because of some signaling system not yet understood, some genes in the DNA of the cells are turned off, no longer needed, and others are turned on. In that way, one cell can become a liver cell with all of its functions, whereas another can become a muscle cell with its obviously different functions. Along this pathway from embryonic stem cell to mature liver or muscle cell are the adult stem cells.

Beginning in 1998, researchers "cultured" human embryonic stem cells in the laboratory. This means that they can be put into a dish with special fluids and cells so that they will continuously divide. Then, so the theory goes, if the fluids are adjusted with certain compounds, they will begin to mature into a specific type of cell, such as a pancreas islet cell that makes insulin.

ADULT STEM CELLS

Adult Stem Cells: What are they? What can they do? Each tissue has a population of cells that can divide as needed to keep the organ or tissue functional as cells die or are injured. We see this with our skin as it constantly lays down new cells that make their way to the surface as the dead cells are rubbed off in the bath or shower.

We also see it when we cut ourselves and in a few days the wound is completely healed. Those were stem cells at work. It appears that essentially every organ has its own pool of such cells. It had been thought that these cells could only repopulate their own organ and that no other source of stems cells existed. But now we know that cells in the bone marrow and perhaps other organs can become stem cells for many different tissues.

The bone marrow makes a lot of precursor cells, including *endothelial stem cells* (the cells that line our blood vessels.) When the inside of a blood vessel is damaged, a signal not yet understood goes to the bone marrow, and some of these cells are released. They home right into the area where the vessel is damaged and assist in its repair. We can find them and count them in the bloodstream. There are fewer present as we age. There are fewer present in patients with diabetes. We might assume that the level in the bloodstream relates to how well or how fast the body can repair itself. Perhaps it also relates to how well the heart can be repaired after damage. What is clear is that lower levels are inversely related to cardiovascular outcomes.

Adult Stem Cells

- Found in Many Organs and Tissues
- Will Divide Multiple Times in Tissue Culture but Not Do so Indefinitely as Embryonic Stem Cells
- Generally Can Only Develop into Cells of That Organ or Tissue
- Some Stem Cells Can Become Cells of Other Organs (e.g., Bone Marrow Stem Cells Can Produce Cells of Many Organ Types such as Heart and Liver)

Osteoblast precursor cells are cells released from the bone marrow that assist in bone repair. They are involved in giving strength and density to our bones. They are present in higher numbers in the bloodstream during puberty when our bones are maturing rapidly, and they dramatically increase after a fracture. If we can learn how these cells are called into action and how they function normally, then it may be possible to figure out how to use them to assist in disease repair. But there is a lot to learn about their basic biology, and it will take years before they are well understood.

The islet cells of the pancreas regenerate themselves. Apparently there is a 1 to 3 percent turnover per day in adults, so it is a very dynamic process. During pregnancy, the number of islet cells increases by 30 to 50 percent. It is assumed that there are stem cells in the pancreatic duct that under the proper stimuli can bud off and make new islet cells. But so far, no one has figured out how to harness this function for the benefit of those with diabetes.

Finally, the precursors of fat cells can differentiate into a variety of tissue types. Could it be possible that a source of stem cells could be fat cells? If so, then there is a ready supply—too many of us have plenty of fat cells.

EMBRYONIC STEM CELLS

It is important to understand just where these cells come from. Those used in science are the result of *in vitro fertilization* (IVF)—that earlier revolution that began in 1977 and that allows an infertile couple to have a child. In this process there are often "leftover" embryos that are otherwise discarded. It is important to understand this point.

With IVF technology, the woman first takes some medicines to stimulate her ovaries to produce multiple eggs in one month—the ovary normally produces one egg at a time. Then the obstetrician obtains the eggs from the woman's ovaries through a large needlelike device inserted into the abdomen via the vagina.

Embryonic Stem Cells

- Obtained From Discarded Blastocyst Cells From In Vitro Fertilization
- Cells Placed in a Tissue Culture Dish with Nutrient Fluids and "Feeder Cells" From Mice
- Cells Continuously Divide as Stem Cells
- Cells Can Then Be Coaxed to Become Cells of Any Body Tissue or Organ

This is relatively safe and painless, but like any procedure, it has its risks. Each egg, along with sperm, is placed into a separate dish with special fluids that give nourishment. Each egg is fertilized by a sperm, and it starts to divide: one cell becomes two, two become four, four become eight, eight become sixteen, and so on. After two days, about thirty-two or so cells—in a mass the size of a pinhead—are in the dish. This is the *blastocyst*.

To be successful with in vitro fertilization, obstetricians have learned from trial and error that they need to put four or five blastocysts into the woman's uterus in order to have one, and sometimes more, grow into a fetus. So the doctor looks at each blastocyst with a microscope and picks the ones that appear to have developed the best. The remainder are frozen.

Even in the best of circumstances only about two-thirds of women become pregnant after four or five blastocysts are implanted. So rather than going through the whole process again, the frozen blastocysts (embryos) can be thawed and tried next time around. If the woman does become pregnant and does not want to have another child, then these frozen embryos can be discarded. It is these discarded embryos that, instead of being dumped out, could be used for extracting stem cells. Roughly four hundred thousand spare blastocysts are available at IVF clinics.

In 1998, scientists under the leadership of Dr. James Thomson at the University of Wisconsin learned how to take some of the cells from these about-to-be discarded embryos and put them into what is called a cell culture—basically a fluid in which the cells can grow to produce more cells.[1] These cells in turn can then be directed to grow into heart or lung or pancreas or other types of cells by using various additives in the fluid in which they're growing. It is from these discards that embryonic stem cells are available to us. Just to be clear: The blastocyst with its thirty-two or so cells is not grown in the culture dish. The individual cells are removed and allowed to divide and grow. These are the embryonic stem cells. But no embryo is growing, just individual cells.

Nuclear Transfer

- Human Egg (Ovum) Obtained from Woman's Ovary Using Process Akin to In Vitro Fertilization Egg Collection
- Nucleus Removed
- Cell Obtained from Patient by Biopsy (e.g., Skin). Nucleus Removed
- Patient Cell's Nucleus Inserted Into Nucleus-Free Ovum
- Ovum Now Acts Like Stem Cell and Will Divide Continuously
- Stem Cells Can Be Coaxed Into Adult Body Tissue
- Tissue Can Be Implanted Into Patient
- Cells Will Not Be Rejected as "Foreign" Since They Carry Patient's Own DNA from Nucleus

NUCLEAR TRANSFER STEM CELLS

A variant of the embryonic stem cell worth knowing about is produced by a process called *nuclear transfer*. Basically, an unfertilized egg is obtained from a woman's ovary similar to the way they are obtained for in vitro fertilization. The egg's nucleus is extracted by a micropipette and then the nucleus of an adult cell is inserted in its place.

This nucleus might be obtained from a skin cell taken from the arm of a patient with a particular problem, such as diabetes. The newly created cell is placed in a culture and with the appropriate signals begins to act like an embryonic stem cell in that it will divide and replicate itself. The hope is that these cells, genetically identical to the patient who had the skin biopsy, could be grown into a vast number of, in this example, pancreatic islet cells and used to treat the patient's diabetes. Since the cells are genetically identical to those of the patient, then his or her body will not try to reject them as if they were "foreigners" that did not belong. This concept is all about personalized medicine.

AMNIOTIC-FLUID DERIVED STEM CELLS

In January 2007, researchers at Wake Forest University School of Medicine reported that they could obtain a form of stem cell from amniotic fluid. The cells grow rapidly in tissue culture and self replicate and can be coaxed to produce fat, bone, muscle, nerve, liver, and blood vessel cells. They seem to be a unique form of stem cells—easily obtained and without ethical controversy.

MAJOR OBSTACLES TO OVERCOME ON THE ROAD TO STEM CELL THERAPIES

The first step, of course, is to have a ready supply of stem cells available, be they embryonic or adult in origin and whether or not they are the result of nuclear transfer. Progress has been made, but the steps are still laborious and complex. Time will help scientists better understand turning on or off the needed genes in the DNA and the chemicals produced by them or other cells that make stem cells divide and persist as stem cells.

Then scientists need to figure out how to prod these stem cells to differentiate into the desired type of cell—islet cell, heart muscle cell, brain cell, and so forth. Much less is known about these requirements, but work is under way. If stem cells are transplanted into a patient, will they be rejected as foreign? Maybe not, but if so, then the nuclear transfer concept should be able to overcome this problem. Remember that an organ or tissue or just an infusion of cells is rejected if powerful drugs are not used to prevent the body from trying to eliminate the foreign tissue.

Islet cells injected into the vein of the liver seem to know to go to the liver and live there and do their work. Also, bone marrow stem cells when injected by vein seem to know to go to the bone marrow, take up residence, and repopulate the marrow of the patient with leukemia, whose own cells were eliminated by aggressive treatment. But would all stem cells know where to go or what to do? Would they go to the heart after a heart attack, or do they need to be infused directly into the coronary arteries or injected into the heart muscle itself? And will stem cells, or stem cells prompted to develop into brain cells, need to be injected directly into those areas of the brain damaged by Parkinson's or Alzheimer's diseases?

Time and experimentation will give the answers. But questions like these should alert you to appreciate that treatment with stem cells—although I am convinced that they represent a major promise for the future—is a future that may still be many years away. Be patient. But while we wait, keep tuned in to the progress that will be made every year.

TISSUE REPAIR

Heart Attack. A lot of work has focused on heart attacks, and it's no wonder when you consider that they are still the leading cause of death in our country and in most of the industrialized world. Heart attacks also cause the heart to pump less effectively—congestive heart failure—because the muscle has been damaged and doesn't have the "oomph" it needs. About four hundred thousand new patients are diagnosed with heart failure every year in the United States. Good drugs and other therapies are available, but the damaged muscle is still damaged. Could it be fixed? Could stem cells repopulate the muscle fibers and divide over and over and differentiate into new muscle fibers or perhaps the small vessels that carry blood to the muscle cells? So far, some exciting animal studies and even some trials in patients are encouraging enough to warrant further testing.

Something, I call it a *homing process,* attracts stem cells to the site of injury, possibly the release of chemical signals that attract the stem cells. But what is the best way to provide stem cells from outside the body or to increase the body's natural production? One method being studied in animals is the use of drugs to stimulate the bone marrow's stem cells to replicate much more rapidly, then circulate in the blood and home in to the injured areas of the heart.

One can take bone marrow stem cells from mice and inject them into the heart along the margins of an experimentally induced heart attack (infarcted muscle). The cells have been found to migrate to the border region around the damaged muscle and convert into heart muscle cells and heart lining cells (*myocytes* and *endothelial cells,* respectively).

Another approach uses a cardiac catheter to inject stem cells into the bloodstream of the arteries of the heart where they then flow to the damaged area. This is less invasive, yet gets the cells to the site of damage in high concentration.

One could also simply inject the stem cells through a vein and hope that they will home in to the heart's damaged areas. Of course, they could just as well go to other areas of the body since they are circulating in the blood in general, but perhaps the signals from the damaged area of the heart are sufficient to attract the stem cells to come and help.

The same approaches have been used in patients, mostly in preliminary, but interesting, concept-testing studies. These are early studies, not ready for generalized clinical care. Large scale clinical trials will be needed to define what works and what does not.

Some patients have had stem cells injected around the damaged area during coronary artery bypass graft, as with the mice. Doctors could demonstrate in some of these patients that the cells engrafted, blood flow increased in those areas, and new "collateral" blood vessels formed.

Often patients who need a heart transplant have to wait more than six months, so they are placed on a heart assist device to help tide them over. At the University of Pittsburgh Medical Center, patients participating in a study receive injections of stem cells from their own blood. Frankly, the doctors are not expecting the infused stem cells to do much to help these critically ill individuals. But when a transplant becomes available, they will be able to study the removed heart and find out where the stem cells went and what they did. Did they become muscle fibers? Did they become blood vessel cells? Did they multiply in the heart? Important questions.

In another study organized by the Arizona Heart Institute and including multiple centers, physicians are collecting skeletal (leg) muscle cells by biopsy. These cells are placed into a culture to allow them to divide eleven to thirteen times and are then frozen until needed. (Think about dividing eleven to thirteen times. If you start with one cell, after ten divisions, you have 1,024 cells; after eleven divisions, you have 2,048 cells; and by thirteen divisions, you have 8192 cells. And you started with many cells, not just one.)

When the patient then has open-heart surgery for either coronary artery bypass or to insert a left ventricular assist device as a bridge to transplantation, the stem cells are thawed and injected into and around the area damaged by the previous heart attack. PET scans which detect molecular activity in tissues done later showed new areas of glucose uptake within the scar area, suggesting that the new cells have "taken" and are active.

Echocardiograms used to study the patients reveal that their hearts' outputs have substantially increased—from 28 to 35 percent after one year. Six of these patients later had heart transplants; in four of them, it was possible to find the skeletal muscle cells in place in the area of injection.[2]

In one study of patients who had experienced a heart attack, *angioplasty* (opening the artery with a balloon) and *stenting* (inserting a wire mesh to keep the artery open) were done immediately after admission. Then they received a drug to boost bone marrow stem cell release into the blood. These stem cells were obtained and placed in the coronary artery inside the stent with a catheter. Heart function at six months improved, especially at the area of the infarct and infusion of cells. There were no "control" patients, so no comparison was done, but the study was important in demonstrating that the procedure could be done safely and quickly.[3, 4]

In another study, doctors gave stem cells through the same catheter that was being used for angioplasty balloon dilatation of the clogged artery. When reevaluated months later, the patients who got the stem cells had, in general, smaller infarct sizes and better heart pumping and better blood flow to that area than did similar patients who had the angioplasty but not the stem cell infusion.

Another study looked at patients who received or did not receive stem cells at the time of infarct. MRI revealed that heart muscle function improved in those who received the stem cells. In general, the early studies suggested that infusing stem cells via a catheter was safe and might well show some improvement in heart function.[5] This led to larger randomized controlled trials.

As of this writing, five randomized controlled trials have been completed and published after careful review. Some have interesting names like "BOOST" or "REPAIR-AMI." In each of the five trials, cells were obtained from the bone marrow, or sometimes from the blood, and infused through a catheter placed into the coronary artery near the area of major damage from the heart attack. Most studies were done shortly after a heart attack occurred; one was done six or more months after a heart attack. The idea in each was to determine if giving these cells—not definitively proven to be stem cells—would improve heart function.

One study found no improvement in heart function, others found some real improvement, but none found really major improvements. Some observations were that it was best to use cells from the bone marrow and not the peripheral blood, perhaps because the cells from the peripheral blood were obtained from small samples and therefore had limited numbers of the needed progenitor cells. It was also better to give the cells a few days after the patient was admitted and treated with angioplasty and stenting, perhaps letting the heart rest a bit before adding in the presumed stem cells. And the responses were better for patients who had the greatest amount of damage as measured by heart function.[6]

This is all exciting, but we do not need to go overboard yet. These were generally small and preliminary studies. The improvements seen have been interesting yet modest. Whether the benefit will be long lasting is not known, but it is enough to encourage scientists and patients to want to go further.

Bladder Control. About seventeen million Americans have bladder problems (incontinence). Prostate surgery, pregnancies, or just aging weaken the muscles that control the bladder opening. Ongoing studies are trying to build up that muscle, called a *sphincter* muscle. Muscle cells are obtained from a tiny leg biopsy about the size of a pea; the stem cells are isolated and grown in a culture until they number about twenty million after a few weeks. These are injected into the weak sphincter muscle in hopes of regenerating it. Will it work? I don't know, but it is certainly intriguing. And by the time you read this, the investigators may have published some results.

Another approach to rebuilding the bladder looks at *tissue engineering,* a concept that may not use actual stem cells but cells further along the path of differentiation. Briefly, a biopsy of the bladder obtains cells. The cells are separated into the two types of tissues in the bladder, the lining cells and the muscle cells. These are grown in the laboratory on a scaffold made of a biodegradable material. The cells growing on the scaffold are fed nutrients so that the cells will grow and proliferate, and somehow they self-assemble on the scaffold. Once it has developed sufficiently, the two layers of cells with its scaffold are surgically implanted in the bladders of children born with deficient bladders. The implanted section has no blood or nervous supply, so it is assumed (or hoped) that these will grow into the cell mass after it is implanted.

Remarkably, bladder function improved in the few children who have had this procedure at Wake Forest Medical Center. It is not certain that these are stem cells as we have defined them, but some of the cells removed at the time of biopsy have been able to multiply and form into a new tissue. So whatever the proper terminology, this type of tissue engineering is exciting and holds some promise for the future. Remember that this is not the same as creating a whole new organ, but it is an early proof of the principle that cells can be taken and grown outside the body and then reimplanted in a useful format. And if stem cells from umbilical cord blood or another source were available, perhaps they, too, could be grown on such scaffolds.

Pancreas Transplant/Islet Cell Transplant. Consider Roberta Gardner, a sixty-two-year-old with diabetes. It started in her late twenties, and she has been taking insulin for more than thirty years. She is the perfect patient. First, she understands her disease and how to care for herself. She eats carefully, she exercises regularly, her weight is just right. She has learned how to adjust her insulin doses to compensate for food, exercise, and rest; and she checks her blood sugar levels with a finger stick multiple times a day.

Even when she wakes up at night, she checks just to be sure her sugar level has not dropped too low. If it has, she will eat some cereal or drink some juice before going back to sleep. But sometimes her sugar drops in the middle of the night, she is not aware, and her husband cannot wake her up. So he calls 911; the EMTs arrive and give her an IV injection of sugar water and now she wakes up—"What happened? Why are these guys here?"

Even with superb attention to detail, she can have a major problem. In part, she has lost her *glycemic awareness* or the ability to sense when her sugar is too low. So her husband often sets an alarm clock so that he can wake up and make sure she is okay. They make it work, but it is tough. In the future, she may benefit from one of the new devices that can continuously monitor a person's blood sugar level and relay the information back to a pump that can give the right amount of insulin. Better still would be a transplant of new islet cells to replace those destroyed years ago by her body.

What about adult stem cells to repopulate the diabetic pancreas? So far this has been disappointing. No one has been able to get adult stem cells from the blood or bone marrow to improve pancreas islet cell numbers or function. The assumption is that it will require embryonic stem cells to cure diabetes.

Consider what happened to a patient I met at our medical center a few years ago. Like Roberta, she had lost some of her glucose awareness but to a much greater degree. She could be driving and suddenly start to fall asleep because of low sugar levels. She was the ideal candidate for a pancreas transplant. But to transplant a pancreas is to transplant a load of potential problems. She became a candidate for a new approach—transplant just the islet cells.

When a pancreas became available, her doctors took the pancreas and "digested" it so that they could extract just the islet cells, and then infused those cells into her vein. From there, those cells "set up shop" in her liver, where they made insulin, detected blood sugar levels, and regulated them properly and naturally. She was much improved and was excited at how much less insulin she now needed and how easy it was to control her diabetes. But the transplant did not have enough islet cells to make her totally insulin- or problem-free. So she got a second transplant and even better control.

She said it was like a "new lease on life—I can do things and go places that I just couldn't do before." Unfortunately, after a few years, many of the islet cells were rejected, and she was back to where she had been with insulin and difficulty controlling her blood sugar. What she needs is an unending supply of islet cells so that if they are rejected over time, she can get a new infusion.

These islet cells could best come from an "islet cell factory," not a cadaver. That is the promise of stem cells. It takes a lot of cells to correct the damage done in diabetes—successful correction requires from two billion to seven billion islet cells. That's why she needed two rounds to get enough from two different cadaver organs. But if stem cells could be grown to produce islet cells, there would be plenty for her and everyone else that needed them, and she wouldn't have to wait for another person to die so that she could benefit from their islet cells.

Islet Cells on Demand. One day, and I believe it will occur within ten to twenty years, stem cells will be mass-grown into islet cells. They will be ready when the patient needs them. Just give them by vein, and they will home in to where they need to go. If they are created from the process called *nuclear transfer,* they probably will not be rejected because they will be developed to not provoke the immune system. Still, whatever process destroyed their own islet cells years before will probably destroy these cells over time as well, unless new drugs are developed to prevent this cell destruction by the body. But until then, just come back for a new infusion whenever needed—like going to the gas station to refill the tank.

Tissue-Engineered Organs. Some remarkable progress has been made in forming new organs or at least tissues that have the functional properties of an organ. For example, at Wake Forest University, embryonic stem cells were taken from cows and developed into a tissue with structures that resemble those in the kidney. And it takes the blood and extracts urine! Now, it is not a kidney, and it cannot be used to replace a kidney, but it does demonstrate a lot of progress on the path to building new organs.

So far, I have been discussing the "home runs," the hopes for cure of disease or regeneration of organs and tissues. But before this can happen, we need to learn a lot more about how these cells function, how they grow and reproduce—what signals, both internally and externally, trigger certain changes and growth patterns. This will take time and many different researchers' work. And there will be many blind alleys and course corrections, just like in all of medical science. Once the signals are well understood, it should be possible to do many things, such as regenerate limbs.

We know that in an experimental animal fetus, if a limb is cut off at a very early stage, it will still grow back—but not if the limb is severed later in development or during adulthood. The genetic directions, however, are still in each cell. If the signals were known, they could be turned on temporarily so that nature could once again take its course and develop a limb. This is many years away, but we will learn how to do it eventually, because it is "natural."

EMBRYONIC VERSUS ADULT STEM CELLS

Although adult stem cells are showing promise in a variety of studies, the fact is that embryonic stem cells apparently have much more potential to renew themselves continuously and to differentiate into any number of cells and tissue types. Adult stem cells just do not have the same potential—at least not with what we know so far.

No one has any ethical or moral concern about the use of adult stem cells, whereas some certainly feel it is wrong to consider using embryonic stem cells. Despite major advances in adult stem cell research, it still appears that embryonic stem cells are needed for many applications, including diabetes. Let me offer my own opinion. Since in the process of IVF about four hundred thousand blastocysts are on the discard list today, rather than simply discarding them, let the cells be used for medical purposes to create stem cell pools that can be used for individuals with diabetes, Parkinson's, heart attacks, and other diseases. To me it is somewhat akin to a family making the decision to donate a loved one's organs after death. Why waste such a useful potential?

Meanwhile, some new reports indicate that embryonic appearing stem cells can be obtained from amniotic fluid. If confirmed, this will be a noncontroversial source of embryonic stem cells.

CANCER STEM CELLS—THE BAD SIDE OF STEM CELLS

Cancers, like tissues and organs, have stem cells. We usually think of a tumor as uncontrollable and growing wildly. True in part, but only a few cells—the stem cells of the tumor—can keep the tumor growing or allow it to spread to other parts of the body. For example, it has long been known that if a scientist took cells from a tumor, say a breast cancer, and injected them in the thigh of the same animal, a new tumor occurred only if a huge number—more than a million cells—were injected.

Did that mean a tumor can spread only if it dumps a huge number of cells into the bloodstream to go off to a distant area? The answer is no. The tumor has to let go of only a few of the stem cells of the tumor. The cancer stem cells look similar under the microscope, but they are functionally different. And it takes less than a hundred of these cells to produce a tumor, not the million needed if one uses a mixture of all the tumor's cells.

Cancer Stem Cells

- Cancers Have Stem Cells Just Like Organs or Tissues
- Cancer Stem Cells Appear to Be the Cells That Keep the Tumor Growing
- Cancer Stem Cells Are the Cells That Cause Spread or Metastasis to Other Parts of the Body
- Finding, Identifying, Isolating and Then Developing Treatments Targeted at the Cancer Stem Cells May Be the Next Major Advance in Cancer Treatment

Cancer stem cells in acute and chronic leukemia are now fairly well characterized. They tend to be *quiescent,* meaning that unlike the bulk of the tumor, they are not rapidly dividing. They tend not to respond to the usual drugs used for cancer treatment, probably because they do not divide rapidly. And they have the ability to eliminate drugs from themselves; in other words, they are resistant to the drug therapy. Gleevec works well for most people with chronic myelocytic leukemia, but eventually, the disease seems to return and is resistant. Apparently it is the CML stem cell, present in small numbers, that was always resistant, and it produces a new set of tumor cells that are also resistant. Even the new drug *dasatinib,* which was developed for resistant cases and suppresses the CML, probably does not eradicate the stem cells.

WHAT IS IMPORTANT IN CANCER TREATMENT?

The key to treating cancer may be to find and destroy the stem cells. Get them, and the tumor cannot continue to grow. But if these stem cells have unique properties, then they may not respond to the usual drugs used for cancer therapy. Our current chemotherapies may be killing off the bulk of the tumor but leaving the stem cells behind, only to regrow again and recreate the cancer. We need to find these cells, study their unique molecular characteristics, and then design drugs that will effectively finish them off. The answers may not be in yet, but it is now possible to direct the work that needs to be done to find and study these cells. I am encouraged.[7]

Cancer stem cells can now be isolated and grown in special immunodeficient mice. In these mice they can be studied and treatments can be tested. But the key findings to be aware of today are that cancer arises from stem cells and that these stem cells have properties different from those of the bulk of the tumor. Just like a lawn full of dandelions that you clip, they will just come right back unless you dig down and get the root.

STEM CELL MEGATRENDS

Stem Cell "Factories" Will Produce Cells, Tissues, and Organs to Replace or Repair the Damaged or Injured

And

Treatments Aimed at Cancer Stem Cells Will Become Available, Effective, and Much Less Toxic Than Present Day Cancer Chemotherapy

MEGATRENDS RELATED TO STEM CELLS

Stem cells are ushering in the era of regenerative medicine, allowing the creation of cells, tissues, and organs to treat or cure diseases and injuries.

This may fundamentally alter our approach to medical care. It will become personalized medicine where one's own cells are used to obtain the nucleus for nuclear transfer on the path to creating stem cells, and from them tissue cells for organ repair or replacement.

WHAT YOU SHOULD KNOW

Since stem cells potentially will be increasingly important to medical care, you should understand what a stem cell is and generally how adult and embryonic stem cells differ. To reiterate, a stem cell can divide into a new stem cell and also into a cell that is destined to become one of the cells in the body's tissues or organs. Embryonic stem cells are those cells that can develop into any one of the body's nearly two hundred different cell types. In effect, they create the cells, tissues, and organs of our bodies. Adult stem cells are present in many tissues and organs and seem to help repair damage from illness or injury. Given that there is intense debate on the use of embryonic stem cells, you should understand that they are derived from discarded embryonic blastocysts created for infertile couples during the process of in vitro fertilization.

With this knowledge, be aware that adult stem cells are being used today for bone marrow transplants. Adult stem cells also are being studied intensively for such uses as assisting the heart attack patient heal his or her damaged heart muscle. Embryonic stem cells are being equally intensively studied to create pancreatic islet cells to treat patients with Type 1 diabetes, and to create cells to reverse the damage done by Parkinson's disease, among many others. Be aware of the stem cells developed with nuclear transfer. The nucleus of a patient's cell is extracted and placed into an embryonic stem cell, which in turn, had its original nucleus removed. Now the stem cell has the genetic material of the patient and can be used to create cells, such as islet cells, that the patient's body will not reject as foreign—a very personalized form of medicine.

We can expect that in the next ten to fifteen years, we will see huge advances in tissue engineering. Look for your old cells to be used in creating new, young stem cells that can be used to replace tissues, organs, bone marrow, pancreas cells, heart cells, and many more. Regenerative medicine will become a reality.

WHAT YOU CAN DO

Except for bone marrow transplantation for diseases like leukemia, cancers being treated with high-dose chemotherapy, and some individuals with immune disorders, stem cells as therapy are still in their infancy. But if you or someone you love has a disease like diabetes or Parkinson's or heart failure after a heart attack, it will behoove you to watch the newspapers or check out the NIH Web site for advances. I suspect that since there is so much basic science still to be worked out, it will be quite a few years before we will see stem cells being used on any sort of regular basis. But time flies, and the science may unravel more quickly than I surmise, so be on the lookout.

Web Sites to Check Out. Two useful Web pages that explain stem cells succinctly yet clearly are *www.lifesciences.umich.edu/research/featured/basics.html* and *www.nih.gov*. The former, from the University of Michigan, has an excellent brief animated section on each type of stem cell, where they come from, how they are cultured, and how they might be used in treating diseases or injuries. The latter is the National Institutes of Health Web site, which gives access to much of the research being done; it has accurate and up-to-date information—with no hype.

CHAPTER 3

Vaccines—Wider Uses, Easier to Administer, Safer

D o you remember the story of Edward Jenner? Back in the 1700s smallpox was a serious, debilitating disease that often led to death. Jenner noticed that milkmaids rarely, if ever, got smallpox. What they did develop, however, was cowpox, a relatively minor disease, although it did leave pox marks on the hands and sometimes the faces of these young ladies. So he reasoned that maybe having cowpox gave the body some type of defense against the more serious smallpox.

In 1796, to test his theory, Jenner took the fluid from cowpox lesions and used it to inoculate the arm of uninfected individuals. It was a pretty crude system of putting the material from the cowpox lesion on the arm and then taking a needle and scratching or scarifying that area. It worked. And with relatively little change since then, the smallpox vaccine has been very effective.

Indeed, it was used to eradicate smallpox from the world a few decades ago. The common name for cowpox was *vaccinia,* from which our term *vaccine* arises. Jenner was the father of vaccination and in the process discovered a method to stop the epidemic of smallpox, rampant in England at the time.

Later came vaccines for tetanus, diphtheria, pertussis (the DPT shot), polio, the common childhood infections of measles, mumps, and rubella (German measles), and later still, chicken pox and hepatitis B. Vaccines were developed to prevent some types of childhood meningitis like *Hemophilus* and other serious infectious aliments. Vaccines for adults came along as well, such as one for *Pneumococcus* to prevent one type of pneumonia in older adults and the annual influenza shot to prevent the flu. Most recently vaccines for shingles, cervical cancer, and rotavirus have been approved.

If you think about it, vaccines are the most cost effective, specific means of preventing infectious disease. They are cheap, easy to administer, effective, and very safe. What can we expect in the coming years? No more shots! Well, not as many shots. Many vaccines will be given by other routes such as by mouth or by skin patches. Usually only one dose of each vaccine will be enough because of the development of new adjuvants.

There will be vaccines for many infections not yet covered, and improved vaccines to replace older ones, that will be more effective and have fewer side effects. Not only infections, but also many chronic diseases from coronary artery disease to multiple sclerosis to cancer may be preventable or treatable with vaccines. Indeed, vaccines will become the cornerstone of much of medicine, especially preventive medicine. And in the developing world where infections remain the major cause of death, frequently in infants and young children, vaccines will be the principal means of bringing these diseases under control. And finally, expect to see *designer vaccines,* ones developed for a specific purpose for a specific individual.

THE IMPORTANCE OF VACCINATION

We tend to forget just how important vaccinations are. Here are two examples, one from the industrialized world and one from the developing world that emphasize just how important it is to get the available vaccines and in the proper time frame.

Influenza causes about thirty-six thousand deaths in the USA every year. About 90 percent of deaths occur in those over sixty-five and especially among those over eighty-five. There are more than one hundred thousand hospitalizations because of influenza each year; most of these are also among the elderly.

So it will come as no surprise that those in nursing homes are very susceptible. The close living conditions make spread easy, and the older age of most residents means that they don't respond as well to the vaccine. But the annual influenza shot can protect at least 50 percent, and probably more, and in the process markedly reduce the spread of the infection around the nursing home. So nursing homes need to make a big effort to get everyone, including the staff, vaccinated. But often that does not happen, and influenza takes a major toll—something that does not need to happen.

Polio is a disease that most of us think of as historical. I remember as a child how anxious my parents and their friends were each summer. *Would polio come around our area this year? Should we keep our children at home and not go to the pool?* It was highly feared in the 1940s and early 1950s. It was easily spread from person to person. About twenty thousand were infected each year, mostly children. You may remember the pictures of kids in iron lungs to keep them breathing. There was no cure, just good nursing care and rehabilitation as best as could be done.

Then in 1955 came the vaccine developed by Jonas Salk. It was a miracle. Every kid got his or her shots of this killed virus vaccine. In 1961, Albert Sabin developed the oral vaccine. It is a live but weakened virus that actually infects and can be passed on to others. This helps to create what is called *herd immunity* among an entire population, vaccinated or not.

Polio soon became a rarity in our country, but not in many parts of the developing world, where vaccines were too expensive and the systems were not in place to administer them. So it persisted with other infectious diseases, including malaria, measles, and tuberculosis. This is unfortunate because like smallpox, polio only infects humans, so it could be totally eradicated from the face of the earth if only everyone at risk could be immunized.

Recently in Nigeria, the polio vaccine was no longer used. This was because of suspicions about the West in general and concerns of a contaminated vaccine in particular. The result was as to be expected. A major outbreak of polio occurred and jumped to other countries. Today, polio persists in seven countries including India, Pakistan, and Nigeria. Hopefully, it will be eradicated—and that is possible with the current safe and effective vaccine. In the meantime, be sure your kids or grandkids do get the polio vaccine because if not, they could be exposed if they come into contact with someone from one of these endemic countries harboring infection.

In America there have been recent outbreaks of mumps and of measles. Here is the measles story: A teenager went on a trip to Romania and was exposed to measles. She had never been vaccinated. When she got home, she attended a church event with about five hundred others. At the time, she did not have the measles rash but did have the prodromal symptoms, such as cough.

Some of the church participants also were not vaccinated, primarily because their families were concerned about the presumed risks of vaccination. These were children who were being homeschooled, where the law did not require vaccination as it does in the public schools. Thirty-four individuals became infected; all were church members, except for one health care worker at the hospital. Twelve were hospitalized, and one nearly died.[1] Message: The so-called "minor" childhood infections are not so mild after all; the vaccines work and are safe, but you and your children need to be vaccinated to be protected.

The World Health Organization (WHO) made these estimates of vaccine-preventable deaths in children, in other words, the deaths that could have been prevented if currently available vaccines, which are universally recommended, were used to their fullest potential. 1,000 children died of polio; 4,000 died of diphtheria; 15,000 died of yellow fever; 198,000 died of tetanus; 294,000 died of pertussis; 386,000 died of *Hemophilus* influenza type b (Hib); and 540,000 died of measles. WHO estimates that there were about 600,000 deaths from hepatitis B infection, mostly acquired during childhood.

Then there are the deaths from infections for which there is a vaccine, but which is not yet universally recommended: 716,000 deaths from pneumococci; 402,000 from rotavirus; and 240,000 from human papilloma virus. These are incredible numbers. The point is that these deaths simply do not need to occur; vaccines can prevent them.

NEW AND IMPROVED VACCINES

There are many new vaccines available, and many more are on the way, but let me use the pneumococcal vaccine as an example. The *Pneumococcus*, more properly, *Streptococcus pneumoniae,* is a major cause of pneumonia in older adults. There are many types—*serotypes*—so being infected by one does not make you immune to infection from another type. Only a few types cause most infections, so a vaccine was developed that incorporated the most common types. It has proven very effective in reducing pneumococcal pneumonia in adults.

Children also get infected with pneumococci and develop infections such as pneumonia, meningitis, and middle ear infections *(otitis media).* The adult vaccine did not work well in infants. So within the last six years, the *protein conjugate vaccine* (PCV-7)—with the seven most common serotypes that infect kids—was created for children. The protein conjugate is an approach to get children's immune systems to respond to the vaccine at an early age since these infections are especially common in infants.

After a few years on the market, it has become apparent that it works very well with three key results. First, there has been a marked decrease in infections, especially the very severe ones like bacteremic pneumonia and meningitis. There has been a reduction in the frequency of kids carrying this bacterium in the upper air passages where it can live until it infects or can be spread to someone else. And there has been a marked reduction in strains of pneumococci that are resistant to the common antibiotics. And there is even some evidence that adults are less likely to carry pneumococci in their upper airways if their children have been immunized. In short, this has been a very useful and effective vaccine in reducing an infection that was not only common in infants and children, but also sometimes very serious.

There is also a new vaccine for meningococcal meningitis, a fearful disease that tends to occur in crowded living situations, such as barracks and college dormitories. The new vaccine is a marked improvement on the current vaccine and should not only reduce infection in those immunized, but also reduce nasal carriage of the bacteria so that it cannot be as easily spread from person to person. The idea is to vaccinate preteens (ages eleven to twelve) when they present for their tetanus-diphtheria booster shot, so that they will be protected when they enter high school, college, or the military.

Recently, two vaccines were approved by the FDA for rotavirus, one from Glaxo and one from Merck. Rotavirus is the leading cause of diarrhea-related illness and death in infants and young children in America. Worldwide, some two million kids are hospitalized and six hundred thousand die. A vaccine is crucial to stop this dreaded infection. One was approved in the 1990s, but it had to be withdrawn because some children developed *intussception,* an unusual problem with their intestines. But the new ones do not cause this problem and they are very effective with more than 90 percent of infants and young children protected, and with a reduction of more than 95 percent of hospitalizations and emergency room visits. These vaccines will have a major impact on preventing rotavirus in the years to come.

Another new vaccine is for herpes zoster (shingles). This is a rash with blisters that is often very painful, and even after the rash and blisters disappear, the pain can last for years and be very debilitating. It is caused by the same virus that causes chicken pox. If you had chicken pox as a child or adult, the virus lives dormant in your nerve cells. Then when body immunity is down, it reappears as zoster. It is very common after radiation for Hodgkin's disease, occurs occasionally after surgery, and may occur among individuals getting immunosuppressant drugs for transplants or cancer.

It also occurs for no apparent reason in older individuals. Indeed, about 20 percent of people over the age of sixty will develop it sometime in their lives. In my practice days, I took care of a lot of patients with lymphomas who developed zoster. Initially there was little to do other than prescribe pain meds, good hygiene, and TLC.

The antiviral drug *acyclovir* was developed, and if given at the very first sign of infection, it could ameliorate the rash, blisters, and pain, but not entirely. So a preventive would be very useful. A zoster vaccine has recently been approved by the FDA. Studies showed about a 50 percent reduction in the frequency of zoster among about thirty-eight thousand people over sixty who received the vaccine, compared to those who were not vaccinated. And those who did get zoster had less painful eruptions.[2] Since I am over sixty, I plan to get my shot during my annual exam this year.

Expect to see many more vaccines like these that will, step-by-step, eradicate or at least reduce the toll of infections in both children and adults. The influenza vaccine will become more effective in older people. There will be better vaccines for cholera and other diarrheal diseases. Expect a vaccine for tuberculosis, and many more.

VACCINES FOR THE DEVELOPING WORLD

When we think of vaccines, we need to divide the world into industrialized countries, those with transitional economies, and developing countries. In the developing world, the proportion of the population less than fifteen years old is very high; for example, Mali has about 50 percent of its population under age fifteen compared to about 15 percent in the industrialized countries. This suggests that the emphasis in the developing world should be on preventing infection in the young. In the developing countries, the top four causes of mortality in children less than five years old are pneumonia, diarrhea, malaria, and measles.

Pneumonia is mostly caused by the pneumococcus, *Hemophilus*, and respiratory syncytial virus (RSV)—all infections for which vaccines exist and are in general use in the industrialized world. Diarrhea is frequently caused by rotavirus, shigella, and a type of E. coli called *enterotoxogenic*—meaning that it makes a toxin that affects the intestines. Vaccines exist for rotavirus and are under evaluation for the others.

There is no vaccine for malaria and although it will probably be ten to fifteen years before one is available, its time will come as well. Worldwide there are about five hundred million people of all ages infected and one to three million die each year, so this is a clear priority.

As for measles, there is an excellent vaccine that has essentially eliminated this infection from the industrialized world, but not from the developing world. Humans are the only host, so it can be eradicated if everyone is immunized. The measles vaccine is very effective. Mass immunization stops its spread. But in the developing world, measles is common and death, as noted previously, tops 500,000 per year.

After this announcement, various agencies began mass vaccinations of children nine months and older. This proved to be very effective. But the agencies need to return every few years and vaccinate young children or the outbreak will return. Right now there is work on an aerosolized form of the vaccine. This will be simpler to administer and will be a huge step forward.

A major problem is that the current vaccine is not effective for kids under about nine months of age. The problem is that after a baby reaches about four months of age, the antibodies (immunity) that came from Mom tend to no longer be sufficient for protection, yet there is just enough left to prevent the current vaccine from creating immunity. With Gates Foundation support, both the University of Maryland and John Hopkins University are working to develop a new vaccine that will indeed work for these infants, since they are at real risk for infection. In the industrialized world this is of less concern because our efficient immunization practices give us herd immunity that keeps measles in check, even for those unvaccinated (including infants) should the virus reappear here. Expect to see such a vaccine in the next five years, or maybe even sooner.

VACCINES FOR DISEASES OTHER THAN INFECTION

The exciting news is that there are now two vaccines that prevent cancer. The vaccine for hepatitis B was developed primarily to prevent the infection, but chronic infection with hepatitis B causes *hepatoma,* a form of liver cancer. Since the vaccine prevents hepatitis B, it also prevents hepatoma from this type of hepatitis. (Hepatoma is also caused by hepatitis C, for which a vaccine is needed.)

Human papilloma virus (HPV) causes most cases of cervical cancer. Vaccines have been developed to prevent infection for some of the most prevalent strains of HPV that cause cervical cancer, and in so doing will prevent most cases of cervical cancer. This is an exciting development. It means that cervical cancer can be prevented, both here and in the developing world where it is much more common. In the USA, about ten thousand cases of cervical cancer occur per year, but worldwide it is the second most common cancer among women, with about 500,000 cases and 230,000 deaths annually.

Given that two cancers can be prevented with vaccines, are there other vaccines against other viruses that cause cancer that can be developed as well? During the next ten to fifteen years, there will be other vaccines developed. One may be against *H. pylori*, which causes not only ulcers, but also the majority of stomach cancers. A vaccine is needed for the Epstein-Barr virus that causes mononucleosis and some forms of lymphoma. The virus HTLV-I causes a form of acute leukemia; a vaccine could prevent this killer. A vaccine against HIV would not only stop the epidemic, but would also mean that other cancers would be prevented as well, such as Kaposi's sarcoma. Overall, vaccines will prevent as many as 15 percent of all cancers—possibly even more.

Cancer can be approached by another vaccine methodology, which we might call *vaccine therapy*. The general idea is to take individual immune cells out of the body, mix them with the antigen of interest from the cancer, often in the presence of immune potentiators, and return these immune cells to the body to attack and destroy the remaining cancer. For example, you know that *prostate specific antigen* (PSA) is made by prostate cancers, and so if it starts to rise in the bloodstream after surgery to remove the cancer, it may mean that the cancer has returned. Scientists are taking immune cells from patients and mixing them with a special form of PSA using electroporation, and then reinjecting the immune cells into the patient. The idea is that the immune cells will now attack the cancer cells that are making the PSA.

Here is another approach, this one focused on chronic myelocytic leukemia. You recall from the genomics chapter that CML is caused by two normal genes (BCR and ABL) coming together to create a new but abnormal gene that produces a protein that leads to the leukemia. Researchers are working on a vaccine derived from a portion of the BCR-ABL protein. The body's response to the vaccine attacks the BCR-ABL affected cells, but not normal cells. Preliminary results suggest that there is an immune reaction and the presence of BCR-ABL protein is way down in the bloodstream with fewer CML cells circulating. Time will tell if this vaccine approach will work, but the point is that such a vaccine was developed and is being tested.

There is also a vaccine under development for treating patients with breast cancer who have been treated and no longer have evidence of disease but are at risk for recurrence months or years later. Recall from the genomics chapter the discussion of HER2/neu in some patients with breast cancer. HER2/neu is a protein that apparently serves as a growth factor for some breast cancers. When it is present in the tumor sample, many physicians will treat the patient with the drug *Herceptin*, which targets the HER2/neu receptor.

An experimental vaccine has been created that attacks this growth factor. It could mean that a woman could be vaccinated instead of taking a drug for an indefinite time period. So far, the vaccine has led to immunity in that the patients developed cells that would destroy the tumor cells. Early results suggested that recurrences are fewer in the vaccinated group compared to the unvaccinated patients, but larger studies will be needed for confirmation.

Other vaccines against cancer will follow.

There is work under way for a vaccine for Alzheimer's. The first vaccine did not work out, but the important point is that a reasonable concept was developed and tested. There is now a promising report of a mouse study. Part of the problem in Alzheimer's is the deposition in the brain of a protein called *beta-amyloid* or Aβ; this also occurs in a mouse model of this disease. Researchers have developed a DNA vaccine against part of the Aβ protein. Compared to the untreated mice, the vaccinated mice developed many fewer amyloid deposits.[3] Be aware, however, that it will be some time before this is fully tested in people and there is controversy as to the importance of the Aβ in the causation of Alzheimer's. For sure, other vaccines will follow.

Two types of vaccines are also being developed to try to prevent atherosclerosis.

The first relates to the concept that the microorganism *chlamydia* may be of importance in the development of atherosclerosis. Chlamydia are known to cause a variety of diseases, including a form of blindness called *trachoma* and pelvic inflammatory disease—and with it infertility or ectopic pregnancies. It is not certain that chlamydia are responsible for some aspect of atherosclerosis but there is evidence that they may be.

Because chlamydia can be eradicated with certain antibiotics, studies have been done using antibiotics given long term to see if they would reduce atherosclerosis, but those studies did not pan out. Preventing infection is different from trying to eradicate it after it may have begun a process of chronic changes. Atherosclerosis is a multifaceted disease and has many elements to its causation including genetics, cholesterol, and diet. But perhaps a vaccine against chlamydia would have an impact. There are no vaccines for chlamydia at present, but there is effort under way to create them. It is reasonable to assume a vaccine will be available in a few years, but then it will take more years to determine if it has any protective effect. The prospect is intriguing.

The other approach is to develop a vaccine to address the deposition of lipids in the arteries. A few research groups have developed vaccines and some have shown a reduction in atherosclerosis in a rabbit model, along with the ability of the vaccine to induce immunity in humans. But no pharmaceutical company has decided to pursue its development. Why? Concern about lawsuits. This is like the situation with the vaccine that was developed for Lyme disease, an infection caused by tick bites that causes many chronic problems if not treated promptly.

The vaccine was proven to be safe and effective and was released by the FDA in 1998. It was removed from the market by its manufacturer a few years later, citing limited sales. More likely the reason was related to lawsuits by some recipients who believed they had been harmed by the vaccine. There is a law that protects the vaccine manufacturers from lawsuits for approved vaccines administered as part of the CDC recommended vaccines for children, but not for all other vaccines. Juries often find for patients over the manufacturer. The company probably decided it was easiest to just withdraw the vaccine rather than continuously fight it out in the courts. Now there is no vaccine for Lyme disease, which is a pity because it is a real problem infection of consequence. And right now there is no progress on the possible vaccine for atherosclerosis.

A very exciting approach with vaccines is to create immune tolerance so that the body will not react against itself and create diseases like diabetes, multiple sclerosis, and rheumatoid arthritis. There are clinical trials ongoing for vaccines aimed at each of these diseases. The idea is not to prevent the disease so much as to slow its progress once it has been diagnosed. Creating immune tolerance is a difficult proposition, and when one element of the immune system is manipulated, it often leads to other changes, also unwanted. But progress is clear. We should know the results in a few more years.

Remarkably, there are even studies ongoing to develop vaccines to aid in breaking addiction to tobacco and cocaine. I would not have even thought of such studies a few years ago, but it just points out the fertile minds of clinician-researchers. who when confronted with a clinical problem, seek out an approach and then work to perfect it.

BIOTERRORISM

I remember talking to our staff about the possibility of bioterrorism in the 1990s before and after I became CEO of our medical center. I wondered what would happen if someone came into the ER and said he had opened an envelope and it was full of a fine white powder. Would the staff know what to do? Who to call? Or would they just take him out into the parking lot in the back and hose him down? So we set up a task force to look at preparedness. But truthfully, the group did not put this assignment high on their overall priority list until 9/11. At a board of directors meeting a few weeks later, I presented a brief slideshow of what the likely "bugs" were that could be used by bioter-rorists. I mentioned smallpox, anthrax, and a few others. It was only a short time later when the anthrax episode occurred.

Anthrax is a deadly infection. There are antibiotics that are effective, but the problem is that many patients only get to a doctor after the infection has developed in the lung and released its toxin.

The toxin is the killer, and there is no good treatment. Once again, vac-cination at least for those at greatest risk, such as the military, makes sense. New vaccines have been developed, one by Human Genome Science, using some of the genomic approaches discussed in Chapter 1.

Those of you who are age forty or older got your smallpox vaccination as a child—and you have that little round scar on your arm to prove it. Smallpox was eradicated throughout the world, and so beginning in 1973, no one in the United States has been vaccinated against smallpox. After smallpox was eradicated, the virus was saved in two secure locations, one at the CDC in Atlanta, Georgia, and one in Moscow. There has been some con-cern that security for the Russian-stored material was breached and it has become available on the black market. Or that somehow others stored some before the final eradication. So possibly smallpox could become a bioterror-ist weapon with devastating results.

That is why the president recommended in 2002 that all health care workers who would be first responders should be vaccinated against smallpox, as should all military personnel. The vaccinations began using *DryVax,* the same vaccine that had been used in the past. But fairly quickly some people suffered quite serious side effects. Actually, this had been known from the pre-1973 experience with the smallpox vaccination. But this time, particularly good records were kept, since now the vaccination was being given as a pro-tection against a risk that was perceived to be real, but certainly not definite. In the past, smallpox—a very real disease—killed a large proportion of those who became infected. So records were kept, and the side effects were carefully studied. If we had an actual outbreak of smallpox, you probably would not hesitate to get the smallpox vaccination. But for a risk of relatively low likeli-hood, the side effects began to outweigh the benefits.

Here are the results. Over about six months, slightly more than 450,000 military personnel were vaccinated; about 70 percent for the first time and 30 percent as revaccination after many years. There were some relatively mild and expected side effects, but the surprise and concern was that thirty-seven people developed *myopericarditis,* or inflammation of the heart. And some cases were quite serious. All of these were among those getting the vaccine for the first time, so it meant a risk of 1 for every 12,819 military people vaccinated.

In early 2003, during the same period, 38,257 civilians, who would be health-care first responders should a bioterrorist attack occur, were vaccinated. There were twenty-two cases of myopericarditis in this group, or seven times the rate in the military group. No one knows why the differences existed between military and civilians, and no one knows why the heart inflammations occurred at all. As word of this got around, civilians stopped getting vaccinated and eventually the program was ended.

The real message is that we need some new approaches to smallpox vaccination that produce good protection, but with much greater safety. The NIH has contracted a number of companies to develop new vaccines that will be both safe and effective. One way to do this is to avoid using living germs, such as the virus—recall that it is not smallpox virus, but its close cousin in the vaccine—used in the smallpox vaccine, or even the killed virus used in the influenza vaccine. What if instead, we used some of the DNA from the organisms as our vaccine? The individual genes from the smallpox DNA, once inside the appropriate cell, would make their respective proteins and those proteins would be presented to our immunity-developing cells, which would then make the appropriate antibody that would defend against that infection.

The problem is that DNA does not get into cells very easily. So if you injected some of the DNA of smallpox or the DNA of the influenza virus it is not likely that much of that DNA would get into cells, and therefore not likely that much immunity would develop.

Electroporation, another approach, combines engineering and biology. The idea is that by putting an electric field around a cell, it will create "pores" in the cell membrane allowing the DNA to enter. The electrical field is turned off (in actual practice it is only turned on for a few milliseconds), and the cells "heal" their cell membrane.

Now the DNA is inside, and it can do its work. I am on the board of Cytopulse Sciences, a company investigating the use of electroporation to assist in DNA vaccination. So far, they have had quite good results in studies with mice and some initial positive findings in studies with monkeys. They have been investigating DNA vaccines for smallpox, Marburg virus, hepatitis B virus, and for dengue virus, all in collaboration with either the Walter Reed Army Institute of Research or the Army Medical Research Institute of Infectious Diseases, where the DNA segments have been developed. And they have been using electroporation with their collaborators to develop the PSA vaccine I mentioned earlier. Only time will tell whether this technology will prove valuable for preventing human disease, but the idea of using DNA rather than the complete bacteria or virus—killed or not—is intriguing.

VACCINE CONTROVERSIES

An unfortunate outcome of vaccine success against the common childhood diseases is a population of mothers who have never seen or experienced the traumas of measles, mumps, rubella, chicken pox, polio, and others. There are "conspiracy theorists" that are certain the government and pharmaceutical industry are keeping critical information hidden, and through popular magazines and Web sites suggest to mothers that vaccines cause diseases such as autism or that multiple vaccines will create "immune overload." Although the possibility that vaccines are causing diseases like autism have been disproven by sound scientific study done by dispassionate experts and that today's vaccines actually include fewer antigens than in years past, many children are still not getting the vaccines that can be of great value. The real problem is that these infections do exist, can cause serious disease, and they are but a plane ride away—as the recent measles importation stresses.[4, 5]

THE MEGATRENDS

For all the children and adults who hate to get shots, the good news is that many vaccines will be given by alternative means within fifteen years. There will be many fewer vaccines by injection. Instead they will be given by nasal spray, by mouth, as a fine mist aerosol, by a "gun" that uses no needles, by tiny pain-free needles, or with a patch on the skin. There will be many new vaccines for infections, some as replacements for old vaccines and some for infections never covered before. New technologies will make vaccines more effective, and highly so, with just one dose—or two at most—with new adjuvants.

Many chronic diseases other than infections will be preventable or treatable by vaccines.

These will include cancers caused by infectious agents and cancers treated with immune modulation. There may be vaccines for atherosclerosis, Alzheimer's, and even addictions. Multiple sclerosis, diabetes, and rheumatoid arthritis—diseases caused in part by the body making an unwanted reaction to normal body elements—may be treated by inducing immune tolerance.

Infections in the developing world, much different from the industrialized world, will begin to come under control with the emphasis on childhood infections. Pneumonia, diarrhea, malaria, and measles are the biggest killers of these children. Vaccines against these infections will be manufactured not by American or European firms, but by corporations in countries like India, where their business model is high volume at low cost.

HIV/AIDS will continue to be a scourge on the world, especially the developing world and those with transitional economies. A vaccine has been elusive, but perhaps in fifteen years or so one will be available.

THE MEGATRENDS

- Fewer Injections — Given Oral, Nasal, Aerosol, Etc.
- Vaccines For
  - Replacement Of Older Vaccines
  - Infections Never Before Preventable
- New Adjuvants Will Mean Just One Dose
- Vaccines To Prevent Cancer
  - Hepatoma
  - Cervical Cancer
  - Many Lymphomas And Some Leukemias
  - Stomach Cancer
- Vaccines To Treat Cancer
  - To Eradicate Remaining Microscopic Disease
- Vaccines To Prevent Chronic Diseases
  - Atherosclerosis
  - Alzheimer's Disease
- Vaccines To Treat Chronic Diseases With Immune Tolerance
  - Diabetes Mellitus Type 1
  - Rheumatoid Arthritis
  - Multiple Sclerosis
- Vaccines For Infections In Developing World Coupled With Effective Immunization Plans
- Vaccine For HIV/AIDS

WHAT YOU SHOULD KNOW

Vaccines have prevented untold numbers of serious infections and death. They are the most effective means available of reducing infection and improving the public health. Be aware of what vaccines are available or will soon be available. Be sure you know what vaccines are available for your children, but don't forget yourself. I will bet you have no idea of when you had your last tetanus or diphtheria shot, and you probably have not focused on whether you have had the pneumococcal or shingles vaccines, available for older adults—more than sixty years old.

Vaccines are generally safe. Even the shot of the influenza vaccine is fairly trivial. And no, it does not cause a minor influenza-like infection with fever and chills and muscle aches, although some do experience soreness at the injection site, and some do have a low-grade fever for a day or two. Some vaccines are more difficult and have more side effects, especially some of those recommended for travel to certain areas of the developing world. But the vast majority of those used for the standard childhood immunizations and those for adult infection prevention are pretty innocuous, while at the same time very effective. And there is absolutely no evidence that any of the childhood vaccines will cause problems like autism.

WHAT YOU CAN DO

Check with your physician and look at the Centers for Disease Control Web site for the list of approved and recommended vaccines for both adults and children (www.cdc.gov/nip/publications). And if you travel, check what vaccines you may need for the countries that you will visit.

Make sure your child gets his or her immunizations on time and on schedule. And make sure you do as well. Don't forget that tetanus immunity begins to wear off, and the chicken pox vaccine—if you received it—does not protect against shingles in older age; you need the new vaccine for that. Get your influenza vaccine each year—no excuses! And watch for the development of new vaccines for many chronic diseases like cancer and diabetes. These may have an effect on some of these difficult diseases, just as vaccines have had a dramatic effect on preventing infections.

PART II

From the Engineering and Computational Laboratories

Part II will address the megatrends emanating primarily from the work of engineers, bioengineers, and computer scientists working with clinicians to devise technologies that will fundamentally change how medicine will be practiced during the coming years. I will use examples of current technologies to illustrate points and give suggestions for where the science is going and what we can expect in the coming years.

CHAPTER 4

Imaging—It's Not Just X-rays Anymore

Four megatrends are developing in imaging. One is the ability to peer into our bodies and see anatomy in stunning detail as never before. The second is the developing ability to "see" into our cells and observe their metabolism and chemical actions. These can be done noninvasively and safely. Not all imaging is done in the radiology department anymore, which leads us to our third megatrend—putting procedures once done in the operating room by surgeons in the hands of "interventional radiologists."

Now we can "see" the metabolic changes arising in the brain from meditating, locate the spread of cancer in areas never before addressed, find narrowing of the coronary arteries without doing a cardiac catheterization, and detect abnormalities of a growing fetus extremely early in pregnancy. Aortic aneurysms can be repaired in the imaging suite in an hour, instead of after multiple hours in the operating room and a week or more in the hospital.

Imaging
"It's Not Just X-Rays Anymore"

- **Anatomic Imaging**
  - Routine X-rays
  - CT (or CAT) Scans
  - MRI Scans
  - Ultrasound
- **Interventional Radiology**

- **Molecular Imaging**
  - MRI Spectroscopy
  - Functional MRI
  - PET Scans
  - Optical Imaging
  - Ultrasound
- **Fused Images**
  - PET-CT

One might even say that the new main entrance to the hospital is the barrel of the CT scanner! The fourth megatrend, now mostly established, is the use of digital imaging rather than film. This means the information collected is available for review anywhere, anytime, by anyone who is authorized. The data can be manipulated to create three-dimensional images and in other ways to improve visualization and interpretation. It also means that you easily can have a copy made—and you should always ask for your copy. What can be imaged, how well, and how fast it can be imaged is advancing exceptionally rapidly. In this chapter, I will go over the current state-of-the-art imaging and try to predict what we can expect five to fifteen years out. But predicting is difficult given how fast imaging technology is changing.

Consider what happened when Lisa Worthington, a fifty-four-year-old engineer, felt pain in her chest. She went to the emergency room where a physician took her history, performed a quick examination, and obtained an electrocardiogram. The classic picture of a heart attack is the "type-A" middle-aged male who comes in saying that he has a severe acute pain, which he demonstrates by holding his tightly clenched fist over his chest, and which he says radiates up into his neck and out along his left arm down to his fingertips. He is pale and sweaty; his pulse is up and his blood pressure is down. The electrocardiogram shows the characteristic changes of early damage to the heart muscle.

Mrs. Worthington's pain was more vague (typical in women) and she did not have the other classic findings that I just described. But heart attack was high on the list of concerns for both her and her physician. Usually, a person like Mrs. Worthington is observed in the emergency room and after a few hours the electrocardiogram is repeated to see if the result has changed. Her blood is tested to check for an enzyme that is released from the heart when the muscle is damaged. But all this takes time. She might be in the emergency room three to eight hours before it is clear one way or the other what is happening.

It was time for a new approach, however. Mrs. Worthington was taken across the hall and scanned by one of the new fast helical CAT scanners. A remarkably clear picture of her coronary arteries was available in less than a minute and she was told, much to her relief, that she was not having a heart attack. Not only that, with a CAT scan it was also possible to rule out the other major life-threatening causes of chest pain—such as a pulmonary embolus, a dissecting aortic aneurysm, pneumothorax, pneumonia, and possibly even gall stones, all of this after just a few seconds. So instead of waiting—and worrying—Mrs. Worthington got the one answer she really cared about: she was not having a heart attack. As it turned out, after an additional history and some further studies, acid from her stomach was regurgitating up into her esophagus (acid reflux), causing her pain. Real pain for sure, but not a heart attack; real pain, but very treatable.

ANATOMIC IMAGING

CAT Scans

To understand this revolution in anatomic imaging let's begin with the CAT scan. CAT stands for computerized axial tomography and is often abbreviated as CT scan instead of CAT. Both mean the same thing.

First, consider the lowly chest X-ray. This is most easily done by following what happened to Ruth Hoffman when she arrived to see her internist because of a persistent and chronic cough. She was sixty-three years old, had been a lifelong smoker, and had had an acute infection about two weeks before. She had seen her physician then, who gave her some antibiotics for an acute bronchitis. Although it cleared, she's still coughing.

Her doctor now sends her for a chest X-ray. She stands in front of a large photographic plate and a beam of X-rays is directed though her to the plate, activating it. X-rays mostly pass through the body, but some are stopped by thick muscle, like the heart or bone, like the backbone and the ribs; so these areas will appear white on a developed film. Conversely, the X-rays will easily pass through the lungs with their air spaces and the film will appear dark in those areas.

Imagine now what we are seeing on her X-rays. It is difficult to see for sure but behind the heart there is a mass. Subtle, but an excellent radiologist will see it. Many physicians would miss it. (Figure 4-2 on page 74 shows it marked with some arrows.) Given her age, lack of any past history of tuberculosis, and her smoking history, odds are this is lung cancer. Based on what we can see, it looks as if a surgeon should be able to remove that part of the lung quite easily and potentially cure her.

For years that's exactly what was done. Mrs. Hoffman would have gone to the operating room and a thoracic surgeon would have removed a segment or a lobe of her lung. But all too often, the surgeon would find that the cancer had spread and that the resection could not proceed. The surgery—with all of its inconvenience, pain, and risk—was a waste.

With the advent of the CAT scanner thirty plus years ago, it became possible to do a much better staging of the cancer. In essence, a CAT scan is akin to taking a picture of a very narrow slice of the body. Imagine "slicing" Mrs. Hoffman in two at the level of that mass in her lung. Now tip her upper body upright so you are looking up into her chest at that level. The CAT scan gives us a picture of that cross-section. In fact, Mrs. Hoffman had such a CAT scan done, and it showed a rather large mass behind her heart.

So she indeed has a very substantial cancer quite visible on CAT scanning but easily overlooked on the routine chest X-ray. CAT scanners made a huge difference for situations like this when they were developed. In effect, the CAT scanner took a single slice at a time and repeated, taking slices up and down the body. Many believe that cross-sectional imaging was the most important advance in radiology in the late twentieth century.

Routine X-ray to left; CAT scan to right. Courtesy Charles Waite, MD, University of Maryland School of Medicine.

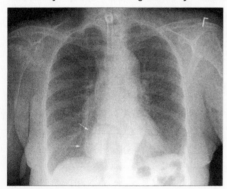
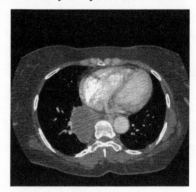

Chest X-Ray   CAT Scan of Chest

In the last few years, as a result of both major engineering developments and vastly improved speed and power of computers, it has been possible to build CAT scanners that can take multiple "slices" at a time. Imagine a CAT scanner that can take eight slices at a time and do a new set of slices every second. In just four seconds, about the length of time you can hold your breath, the CAT scanner could have done thirty-two cross sectional slices of your chest. That provides a lot of information. Because the scanner goes so fast, it allows for greater resolution because there is less distortion from body movement.

Because the computers are so fast, pictures can be evaluated in real time and, most amazingly, converted into three-dimensional images. One can see the outline of the heart or the lung or any other object or organ in the body. It is also possible, again using the digitized information, to create virtual bronchoscopies, colonoscopies, or aortography. The engineering and computational abilities have increased rapidly, so that in just a few years the eight-slice scanner was upgraded to sixteen, then to thirty-two, and now sixty-four with 128 slices and 256 at a time on the near horizon. With these incredible speeds the resolution is even greater. But since so many slices are taken, it does mean that you get a lot more radiation than from a simple chest X-ray.

Too much radiation can increase the risk of having some type of cancer occur twenty, thirty, or more years later. So we want to use this capability appropriately—do it when it will give us important information, but don't use it for "fishing expeditions."

Let's consider how we can put this incredible technology to use. As the patient Lisa Worthington illustrated, it is now possible to get quite excellent pictures of the arteries that go to the heart itself, the coronary arteries. The sixty-four-slice machine gives dramatic pictures of the coronary arteries; a thirty-two-slice machine is pretty good. A quick CAT scan can present the heart's exterior in any orientation or from any side in three dimensions.

Or one can create any cross-section of the heart or a view of any heart valve. Then, it's on to the major blood vessels, the coronary arteries.

The future is virtual as the computer "unpeels" the coronary artery from the heart, straightens it out on the computer screen and allows you to literally peer down the lumen on the monitor. The computer then measures the vessel's cross-sectional diameter at various points and calculates the degree of obstruction or what we call *stenosis*. This is close to what can be done in the cardiac catheterization laboratory with an angiogram—the gold standard today.[1]

I think it is fair to assume that this type of CAT scan will replace the angiogram in the not-too-distant future as the primary test to diagnose obstructions in the coronary arteries. Of course one would still need to go to the cardiac cath lab to have a repair done, such as angioplasty or the insertion of a stent; we will discuss this later.

A regular chest X-ray cannot pick up cancer of the lung until it is at least a centimeter (ten millimeters or about a half an inch) in diameter. That means it's past the state of being curable with surgery, as we saw with Mrs. Hoffman. As a result, regular chest X-rays are no longer used as a screening tool because they are simply not useful. But the CAT scanner can find much smaller lesions, down to about two millimeters in size. Does that mean that lung cancer can be found early enough to be curable?

An ongoing study called the International Early Lung Cancer Action Program (I-ELCAP) now has more than thirty-one thousand patients enrolled who are age sixty or older with a ten-year-plus smoking history.[2] Obviously, these are high-risk individuals. The study centers were both academic and community hospitals using spiral CT scanners beginning in 1993 to screen for lung lesions. As of the time I am writing this, 484 cancers have been found and of those a remarkable 85 percent were found to be stage 1, which means potentially surgically curable. Indeed the estimated ten year survival for these patients is a remarkable 88 percent. An important question is how many individuals in this study had a suspicious finding on their CAT scan that turned out to be benign rather than malignant after evaluation, that is, a false positive. It turned out that forty-three such false positive cases were found based on their screening methodology. You will have to judge if that is an acceptable or unacceptable number of cases where screening led to what ultimately proved to be unnecessary procedures.

This was not a controlled study so we don't know what would have happened to these individuals if they had not been screened but just came to their physicians as usual. To overcome this issue, the NIH is funding such an evaluation now. Time will tell how this will turn out, but I suspect that there is real value here. Lung cancer is usually found when it is far advanced and not curable. The I-ELCAP study stands that notion on its head. Not only that, this study was begun in 1993 using the older types of CAT scanners. With the newer CT technologies, not only will it be possible to get down to a millimeter or maybe even less, but the scanners will differentiate with much greater assurance which abnormalities are truly cancer and which ones are probably not. (We will address this issue further when we look at molecular imaging.)

You may have read about the virtual colonoscopy. Remember that since the CAT scan takes these cross-sectional images and the information is digital, it is possible to use the computer to create a virtual picture of any organ, including the large intestine or colon.

In a routine standard (or optical) colonoscopy, an endoscope is inserted through the anus, then up the rectum and colon all the way to the appendix so that the gastroenterologist can visualize the entire colon. We know that all colon cancers start as a polyp, so even though most polyps do not develop into cancer, the gastroenterologist will remove any polyps that are seen during the colonoscopy procedure. In this way colon cancer can be prevented, or should a small cancer be detected, it also can be removed during the colonoscopy. The result is that many lives are being saved with screening colonoscopies starting at about age fifty, earlier for those with a family history. But as in any procedure there is some risk, and it does require either anesthesia or conscious sedation.

Virtual colonoscopy is done with a CAT scan. It does require before the procedure, as optical colonoscopy does, that one consume a clear liquid diet for twenty-four hours and take a strong laxative to purge the colon. When experienced radiographers perform the procedure—and this is critical—it will pick up more than 90 percent of the polyps or tumors that would have been seen with the optical colonoscopy. It picks up almost all of the larger polyps, the ones most likely to harbor or develop into a cancer. False positives occur only about 4 percent of the time, so although you will need to take a clear diet for twenty-four hours and clean out your bowels, you are spared the discomfort and risk of the actual mechanical colonoscopy. Probably in a few more years virtual colonoscopies won't need the bowel prep. Now that will be a really big advance in comfort!

Most colonoscopies are negative, meaning only about 20 percent of patients will have a polyp. If something is found virtually, you can immediately move down the hall for a regular colonoscopy to remove the polyp. This means that more people might opt to have the procedure done, and only those who truly need the optical colonoscopy will have it, saving time for both patient and gastroenterologist. It is imperative that a skilled radiographer reads these virtual exams, but there are relatively few in the country today. The other critical condition is the guarantee that if something is seen, you will be immediately moved into the GI suite so that you will not have to go through a second bowel preparation.

The message—you should start having a colonoscopy when you turn fifty, sooner if you have a family history of colon cancer. If you should opt for the virtual colonoscopy, be sure that the institution where you have it done has experienced reviewers and an arrangement to send you directly to the GI suite if a polyp is found.

The modern CT scan can help with chest pain diagnosis and can save you the experience of a regular colonoscopy. CT scanning also advances trauma care. One type of CT scanner can go from head to toe in thirty seconds or less looking for injuries from trauma. If something is found, then the machine can zoom in on specific smaller areas for more detailed evaluations. This means that injured patients do not need to be repeatedly moved or manipulated and indeed the scanner is portable, so it can actually come to the bedside. This allows for fast, at-the-bedside triage to decide which injured patients need to go to the regular CAT scanner and who may need to go immediately to the operating room. This can be especially helpful for patients with multiple fractures or chest damage or both. This helps trauma surgeons obtain a quick, accurate injury diagnosis, which is critical in trauma care. It used to take nearly an hour to X-ray all four extremities. Now it can be done in seconds, with multiple views, at the bedside, and since it is digital, the results can be viewed at any location.

Following is another example of how the CT scanner can be helpful with trauma. Someone called the other day to get advice on a friend who does a lot of horseback riding. During the weekend, she slipped and the saddle horn jammed up under her ribs. She continued riding for about an hour, but then decided something was badly wrong and went to the ER. A CAT scan showed that her liver was lacerated (torn) but appeared to have stopped bleeding.

She needed a few units of blood and watchful waiting and returned home after a few days of observation. If the bleeding had continued, the CAT scan would have been repeated, and she would have had a procedure done with a catheter to stop the bleeding. Instead of open surgery, the doctor would have inserted a catheter in the large artery in her groin, passed it up to the artery that goes to the liver, and then gone into the liver to the site of the bleeding. A material would have been injected there to block (embolize) the broken artery(s) to stop the bleeding—a real advance from the open surgery of the past used for both diagnosis and to stop the bleeding. Instead of a prolonged surgical recovery, the bleeding can be stopped and patients can go home in less than a week.

You may not have thought much about autopsies, but they have revealed enormously valuable information over the years.

The virtual autopsy is a new approach. These incredible new CT scanners can look deep into the body and at least determine anatomic changes that may not be realized by routine examination. The military is doing a virtual autopsy on every solider that is killed, and they learn a lot. The soldier can be reconstructed in virtual form from the CT scanner. The wounds can be reconstructed as well. Using inverse prediction techniques, it is possible to understand how the injuries occurred. This allows for scenario planning with feedback to commanders in the field. Reviewing and analyzing all of the data from the virtual autopsies gives commanders the option to change tactics, such as their operational approaches or changes in body armor. The aim is to save more lives through better understanding of the injuries that cause death.

In the chapter on digitization of medical data, I discuss what is known in the military as the PIC, or Personal Information Carrier. Briefly it is a flash memory device—like you find in your digital camera—that is worn as a dog tag. It can hold personal medical information, which is then available to a medic on the battlefield, at the base hospital, or at the major referral hospitals

in Germany or the United States. It is likely that someday all military personnel will have a baseline CT scan done and placed on their PIC. Then any
injury that occurs can be compared to that baseline.

What about the total body scan sites that are popping up at your local
mall? Should you get one to see if there is anything abnormal? I do not advise
it. Everyone's anatomy is somewhat different, so something will undoubtedly
be found. Then you need to decide if it needs to be followed up on. This can
create a lot of anxiety, and it is likely to lead to additional testing, much of which
may not be necessary. I think a better approach is to see your doctor regularly
for a basic examination. Then if the doctor feels an imaging procedure is
needed, get the right one of the specific part of the body and at a good center.

Following is an example of how information from one of these scans can
cause problems. George Ledbetter was in his mid-fifties and in relatively
good health. We have known each other for about twenty years but not as
patient and doctor, although he often asks me for opinions on medical issues.
He does not smoke and he does not drink. His cholesterol level is borderline.
His doctor suggested he lose a few pounds and exercise regularly—both difficult for him.

While attending a conference, he was not feeling well. He used a free
machine at a drugstore to check his blood pressure and found it to be somewhat elevated. He mentioned this to a colleague who said that perhaps it
would be a good idea for him to get a total body scan. When he returned
home, he had one done at a nearby mall. That was when the problems began.
He was told that he had excessive cardiac calcification, which could be a sign
of potential heart problems.

He called me, extremely anxious and agitated. I lined up an excellent cardiologist who agreed to see him the same day. The cardiologist looked at the
report and said, "No, it really does not represent a heart problem." But even
after a thorough examination by the cardiologist, my friend was still concerned. The only way to reassure him was to do an electrocardiogram, a stress
test, and a few other procedures. Finally, it was all completed, and he could
rest assured that he was okay—although he still needed to lose some weight
and get more exercise. Frankly, I think he was more at risk from the acute anxiety that he experienced for a few days than anything else. The moral of my
story is that you may not like what you find, and more importantly, it may
not be relevant.

Do I seem to be giving two separate and competing messages? Not really.
Someday soon it will be appropriate for everyone to have a scan done when they

are, say, eighteen years old. This will be their lifetime baseline scan, and can be kept digitally on a PIC-like device, the way the military does. It can be used for comparison when the person develops a disease or experiences some type of trauma. This is different from going to the mall for a scan "just to see how I am."

I mentioned at the beginning that the information from the CAT scanner is digitized so that it can be reconverted by the computer into any plane or angle that would be helpful to the physician. Recall that it is also possible to create three-dimensional images and rotate them on the computer screen to see an organ from any direction, look inside, and so on. Now consider a surgeon about to do an operation. From the surgeon's perspective, the fewer surprises during surgery, the better. That is exactly what is beginning to happen as a result of these revolutionary changes in imaging ability.

I watched the computer screen recently while I was shown the images from a patient who had a defect in his diaphragm, the big thin muscle that moves our lungs as we breathe. The surgeon wanted to know before surgery as much about that defect as possible. On the computer screen I could see the heart in red, the diaphragm in green, and the stomach in white. The lungs and liver had been deleted for this purpose by the computer.

We could see that the stomach was pushing up through that defect in the diaphragm, right up into the cavity where the left lung sits. We could also see exactly where the spleen was and the kidney and the adrenal gland on that same side. All of this helped the surgeon plan how to go about the surgery. Could he do the entire surgery through an incision in the abdomen or was there a need to also make an incision in the chest wall? Could it be done laparoscopically, less invasively, or was a large open incision needed? The surgeon was delighted to have all this information in advance. It was obviously going to make a big difference in how he approached the surgery for this patient. Personalized medicine.

MRI Scans

Let's turn to the magnetic resonance imaging. Think of MRI—like a CAT scan—as providing anatomical or structural information. But it is also capable of producing functional information. It does not use X-rays, but instead is able to detect the radio frequency changes of hydrogen atoms within strong magnetic fields. These changes can be measured and those measurements can be transformed into an image. MRI is excellent for looking at soft tissue and nervous tissues like the brain or spinal cord. For example, you can see the spinal cord as it rests within the vertebral canal (the channel formed by our backbones to protect the spinal cord). If a disc has slipped and is pushing on the spinal cord, it is easy to see.

Advances on the engineering side of MRI devices include stronger magnets, new approaches to software, and other improvements that either increase resolution or increase the speed at which images can be taken. Exciting new applications include *diffusion imaging,* which can be used to map the brain's fiber tracks and how they have been damaged by strokes and other brain diseases. There is *perfusion imaging* where it is possible to measure the flow of blood in the heart. *Functional imaging* refers to highlighting regions of activity in the brain. Functional MRI (FMRI) has been used to map task-based brain activity in neurological and psychiatric diseases and provides a fascinating understanding of normal brain function. FMRI can map out the areas of the brain critical to speech and movement and the tracts that move that information to other areas of the brain. With this information at hand, surgeons can more accurately resect a brain tumor without causing unwanted side effects from the surgery. Some centers report as much as a fivefold decrease in complications as a result of mapping.

The fourth new area is *peripheral angiography* (literally meaning a graphic representation of a blood vessel), which can be used to pick up aneurysms (balloonlike bulges) in the aorta, the large vessels in the legs, and even in the brain. Finally, there is *spectroscopy,* the way in which MRI detects unique chemical signatures and can combine them with structural imaging. It is proving useful in studying cancer.

The new MRI machines can be used to do many types of cardiac evaluations. Opinions differ as to whether CAT scans or MRI scans will ultimately be more valuable here. I certainly do not know the answer, but what is clear is that both technologies are advancing at ever more rapid rates, and it may well be that MRI will be able to do coronary angiography or see inflamed atherosclerotic plaques in a coronary artery.

Many cancers, such as prostate cancer, have an increased level of a normal body chemical called *choline* relative to normal cells. This can be detected by the MRI spectroscopy technique. In prostate cancer, the MRI spectroscopy can visualize the specific areas of the prostate where the cancer is located. This obviously can be used to help in diagnosis and is particularly useful for treatment planning and guidance when implanting radiation seeds into the prostate.

Functional MRI detects the ebb and flow of blood to the brain. Even marketers are getting into the act. They can look for the ebb and flow of blood to the brain centers of pleasure, thought, or memory. If you like what you are seeing, the blood flow to the prefrontal cortex of the brain increases. That is not exactly the same as hitting a "buy" button, but auto manufacturers, movie studios, and bottled water distributors have all been doing tests to see how their advertising turns on your pleasure centers.

Here is another interesting observation. If you have a functional MRI done, a particular area of the brain lights up if you experience pain, such as a mild electric shock. Those same areas of the brain will light up if you observe your loved one experience the same pain. You did not experience real pain; you experienced empathy and apparently the same part of the brain responds to either real or imagined pain.

MRI is useful for detecting aneurysms in the arteries in the brain. These balloonlike bulges may rupture, spilling blood into the brain, and causing severe damage or death. Unlike the typical stroke caused by a blood clot, the onset of a hemorrhagic stroke is usually foretold by a sudden-onset severe headache. A new, nonoperative technique inserts a catheter into the arteries of the brain, directing it to the aneurysm and placing tiny metal coils that cause the blood to clot—curing the aneurysm. It is critical to fix an aneurysm immediately when a person has symptoms, such as headache.

Does it make sense to be scanned for these aneurysms just like scanning for aortic aneurysms in the abdomen? The latter can be picked up by a simple, cheap ultrasound test. A brain aneurysm requires an expensive MRI for detection. And which aneurysms should be treated? Is there a size that suggests trouble ahead? Evidence suggests a genetic component to the development of brain aneurysms. Perhaps a genomic analysis will become available in a few years. Meanwhile, an ongoing study suggests that those with a strong family history are at greatly increased risk. Such individuals might benefit from being scanned. But still the question remains as to which discovered aneurysms need to be treated and when. Given that a relatively noninvasive technique exists for a cure, this becomes an important question to resolve. A piece of advice: if you or a loved one develops a sudden, very severe headache for no apparent reason, go to the ER immediately and insist on an MRI scan. Don't go home without one—it could save you or your loved one.

Ultrasound

The basics of ultrasound are that the machine sends out high-frequency sound waves that reflect off body structures, like the concept of sonar used by ships. The computer receives these reflected sound waves, converts them to electrical signals and uses them to create a picture. Unlike an X-ray or CT scan, there is no radiation exposure with this type of imaging. So ultrasound is quick, safe, cheap, and simple. It is a useful way of examining many of the body's internal organs, such as the heart, liver, gallbladder, kidneys, and bladder.

Because ultrasound images are captured in real time, they can show movement of internal tissues and organs. They can also enable a physician to see blood flow and heart valve functions. This can help diagnose a variety of heart conditions and assess damage after a heart attack. Some techniques add clarity and functionality to ultrasounds in certain situations. For example, salt water can be agitated in a way that encapsulates some air. Then when injected by vein, it will help enhance the image contrast within the heart or blood vessels.

Ultrasound is used in every obstetrician's office. It can be used to check the fetus's size, the size of the birth canal, and can tell you the sex of your baby. It becomes the first photo of your baby. It can also be used to look for defects such as congenital heart disease. And it can be used to find problems that can be treated in utero with tiny instruments guided by the ultrasound.

Ultrasound is also used in most urologists' offices. They use it to see how much urine might be left in the bladder after voiding. It is accurate down to less than an ounce. Much better than the old method of inserting a catheter!

In the operating room, ultrasound can be used to check the surgery as it proceeds. And it is possible to couple a preoperative MRI or CAT scan with real-time ultrasound. The ultrasound is being used as a translator, asking the computer to show on a monitor one or another angle of the preoperative scan. This allows the surgeon to visualize from any angle the patient's own anatomy as detected on that preoperative scan. These are just two more techniques that help ensure that surgeons will not have surprises in the operating room.

Ultrasound devices have become miniaturized and portable so that they can be used in the emergency room to help with triage in trauma or sports injuries. Walter Griggs was a thirty-four-year-old carpenter who was working as part of a team building a new house. He was using a pneumatic hammer with three-inch nails and somehow lost his balance, pulled the trigger, and a nail was driven directly into the center of his chest. He was quickly brought to the trauma center where he pointed to the head of the nail and said it did not really hurt much. He was scared, of course, so his pulse was elevated, but his blood pressure was good and nothing overt suggested major internal bleeding. But the ultrasound, done immediately and right at the bedside, showed that the nail had punctured directly into his heart and that blood was leaking out of his heart and into the pericardium—the sac that surrounds the heart.

Once enough blood got into the sac, it would begin to constrict the heart, and the heart would not be able to pump enough blood for his body. He was taken immediately to the operating room where the ultrasound was able to continue to monitor where the nail was in relation to the heart and where the surgeons were operating. For Mr. Griggs, the handheld ultrasound essentially saved his life because it was able to immediately show exactly where the nail was and guide the surgeons in the repair.

Ultrasound technology has advanced dramatically and will continue to do so. Since the information collected is digitized, it can be manipulated to create—with the correct equipment—a 3-D image that can be rotated. For example, the heart can be rotated just as though it was in the examiner's hands. Truly beautiful images of the unborn baby can be obtained. Parents can note the resemblance to relatives before birth, and physicians can use this bonding between mother and fetus to encourage smoking, alcohol, or drug cessation. Many fetal anomalies, such as cleft lip/palate, recessed chin, or spinal problems like spina bifida can be detected in fine detail.

In adults and children, heart abnormalities become clear; surgery can be planned. Stomach and gallbladder 3-D imaging can markedly assist the surgeon design the proper approach. And since the data is digitized, it can still be manipulated on the computer after the patient has left, as is done with digitized X-rays such as CT scans.

Molecular Imaging

A radical change for radiology is the development of functional or physiologic imaging instead of just anatomic imaging. Basically, this revolutionary change is aimed at uncovering the "process of disease" rather than the location or shape of disease.

The CT and the MRI scanners ushered in a revolution in radiology a few decades ago, producing superb anatomic images that are rapidly improving. Now we will witness a new revolution—a transformational technology— changing how we understand disease through molecular imaging. In the past the radiographer saw a shape and offered a diagnosis such as "broken bone" or "pneumonia." With molecular imaging, we will "see" what is happening at a molecular level in our cells. Imaging the actual disease process is a radical change, and it will radically alter medicine.

Elements of molecular imaging have been around for some years (we have already discussed MRI spectroscopy and functional MRI), but the acceleration and the new technologies are rather dramatic. The acceleration will only pick up speed in the coming years with increasing numbers of new technologies. Molecular imaging will be able to look at the cellular level of function and the molecular level as well. The key technologies available or in development today are nuclear imaging using PET or SPECT imaging, optical imaging, magnetic imaging with MRI, and ultrasound imaging.

Molecular and Functional Imaging

- PET Scans
- Optical Scans
- SPECT Scans
- Functional MRI Scans
- MRI Spectroscopy
- Ultrasound

PET Scans

PET stands for "positron emission tomography" that—unlike X-rays, CAT scans, or MRI scans—is entirely an image of function not of anatomy. A radioactive pharmaceutical is injected into the vein, hence the term *nuclear* imaging, and then circulates in the blood and goes to various cells. For example, a radioactively tagged glucose (sugar) molecule will go to cells and be taken up and used as energy. Cells that have high metabolic activity will take up more of the radioactive glucose. Radioactivity can be picked up by detectors, which then create an image. In effect we are taking a picture of metabolic activity, whereas most of our other imaging devices are taking a picture of anatomy.

PET has emerged as a powerful imaging tool for cancer and heart care and is increasingly being recognized as valuable in neuro care as well. It is excellent for detecting occult tumors and for staging cancer. Sometimes a patient presents to the physician with a *cancer of unknown origin*. This means that there is cancer in the bone or liver, for example, but it is not obvious where the primary site of that cancer is. PET scan can frequently find that site.

Alternatively, the doctor may know where the primary site is but not know if it has spread. Here again PET scanning is often quite valuable. Sometimes when cancer is treated with radiation or chemotherapy, the X-ray, CAT, or MRI scan still shows something left behind. But is this tumor, or is it scar tissue, fibrous tissue, or just necrotic dead tumor cells? Here again the PET scan can be helpful. The PET scanner can also see changes in a tumor much sooner than can a CAT scan or MRI.

It can give an early yet accurate assessment, which is vital in evaluating treatment. A tumor that shows an early response to a drug suggests that the patient should stay on the current therapy. But another patient whose cancer is not showing a response can be promptly switched without getting repeated courses of chemotherapy to no avail. These early changes seen on PET correlate well with the ultimate response seen after time and multiple courses of cancer chemotherapy.

In studying the heart, PET scan can show whether an area of the heart is being well perfused with blood and also whether the heart muscle has been damaged by lack of blood flow. These changes can be seen quite quickly after the fact, so PET can be a big help in properly analyzing the status of a person's heart function.

PET in Monitoring Therapy of Cancer

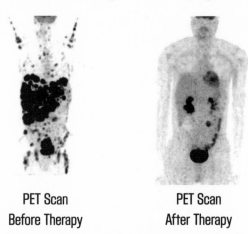

PET Scan
Before Therapy

PET Scan
After Therapy

Courtesy Bruce Line, MD, University of Maryland School of Medicine.

PET can be used to learn who is in the earliest stages of Alzheimer's disease. A molecular marker called Pittsburgh Compound B (PIB) can be injected into a vein, travel to the brain, and then bind to the plaques of beta-amyloid that characterize Alzheimer's. PET scanning will pick up the radioactivity of this agent and show the plaques. It turns out that many people have abnormal scans years before they have any cognitive impairment. Personally, I would not want to know if I am about to start a downhill course from Alzheimer's, since at this time there is nothing to prevent progression. But when treatments do become available, it would allow therapy to begin before irreversible damage occurs.

OTHER APPROACHES TO MOLECULAR IMAGING

The idea of molecular imaging is to get down to the behavior of individual cells and specific molecules within cells. PET scanning technology has been one of the first into this field. Many new biomarkers other than radioactively labeled glucose are becoming available. Agents now can target atherosclerotic plaques, blood clots (thromboses in the coronary arteries, the carotid arteries, or the brain), the damaged brain areas in Alzheimer's disease, and the areas where Parkinson's begins, the changes in arthritis, and the inflammation of infections.

For example, some patients with breast cancer have elevated levels of the growth factor HER2/neu. Using an agent that can bind to HER2/neu, the PET scanner can image this growth factor in the tumor cells. Then it is possible to determine almost immediately how a drug or drug combination affects it. This will offer a rapid understanding of whether a drug is working—another example of the concept of personalized medicine. For this patient, we are able to find out whether a drug is likely to work, and then whether it actually has worked. It is a good technology for both assisting in diagnosis and then assisting and monitoring therapy.

This can be carried even further. Once an agent or probe has been created that will find and bind to the target (like a heat-seeking missile) the binding agent can be constructed to deliver a payload of drugs or biologics that destroy the disease.

PET is proving useful, but MRI and optical imaging, neither of which produces any radiation exposure, may well become the techniques of choice in the future. These will require their own set of new agents that can molecularly target the site of interest and then be detected by MRI or optical imaging scanners. Many have been tested and many more are on the way.

Molecular Imaging with MRI

MRI gives both anatomic information and molecular information at the same time, a big advantage since the doctor will know not only *what* is happening, but also *where* it is happening. Two agents that are used with MRI to get molecular information are gadolinium and iron oxide. Gadolinium is used in mammography, and iron oxide can be used to detect inflammation in a joint, an infection, or an atherosclerotic plaque. Iron oxide has been used to detect small metastases of prostate cancer to the nearby lymph nodes. This is important for establishing the areas to receive radiation therapy. Until now, these tiny lesions would have been missed, and the radiation therapy ports might have been too narrow, allowing the cancer to recur.

Molecular Imaging with Optical Techniques

Optical imaging is a relatively new field that is becoming important, initially in small animal research and increasingly in human settings. An example is to use infrared rays, which can easily penetrate through a mouse. The idea is to attach a near infrared fluorescence agent to a compound that, when injected, seeks out a specific target, such as a tumor. This optical agent fluoresces in infrared light and thus can be detected and shown as an image. Visible light cannot penetrate tissues very far but infrared can penetrate to a fair depth. Detectors can be placed in the body to pick up the signal if it is coming from a deep location.

Here are some examples. A cardiac catheter can be placed in a coronary artery and used to detect fluorescence emitted from an agent that binds to cells in the atherosclerotic plaques. A gastroscope in the stomach can pick up the fluorescence from an agent that has been bound to a stomach cancer. And a detector placed just over the carotid arteries in the neck can detect the inflammatory activity in the plaque in the artery or the new blood clot that has formed over it. Soon there will be agents that can detect the inflammatory activity in an arthritic joint.

Infrared optical scanning also could be used to double-check a surgeon's work. When a surgeon finishes doing a coronary artery bypass graft (CABG) it would be valuable to be able to check out each vessel and make sure the bypasses are working before closing up all the incisions in the chest. A possible approach would be to inject indocyin green into the coronary arteries. The indocyin green, which is safe in the human body, will react when infrared light is shined onto it, so you would get a picture similar to an angiogram. The cardiac surgeon would have a quick, easy, and cheap method to check his or her work, and it would not expose either patient or staff to radiation.

Molecular Imaging with Ultrasound. Ultrasound for molecular imaging is still in its infancy, but it's inexpensive, has good resolution, and combines the molecular information with its intrinsic anatomic data. With newly developed agents that can bind to various cells, ultrasound will become more and more useful to study cancer, the inflammation in atherosclerotic plaques, and blood clots.

Fusing Anatomic and Functional Information

In years to come, molecular imaging will almost always integrate functional information with anatomic images so that we will know both what is happening and where it is happening.

Currently, much molecular imaging is done without the corresponding anatomic image, but this will change as the technology advances in the next few years. PET scanners can be teamed with CAT scanners—two consecutive "barrels" with both scans done sequentially—then the data fused together. In fact, most PET scanners sold today come as combined PET-CT units. This markedly increases the utility of the PET scanner.

PET-CT scanning of the heart, using rubidium as the nuclear agent, can give a quantitative measure of the heart's "flow reserve," the extra we need when we run, bicycle, or carry in the groceries. As an example, a man was tested with the usual SPECT technique and learned that the flow of one of his coronary arteries was limited compared to the other two. SPECT data is relative, using colors to show differences, such as green and blue being worse than yellow and red. But when retested with rubidium PET-CT with its quantitative capability, it was clear that all three arteries were abnormal with one more so than the others.

Instead of angioplasty or surgery, he opted for a rigorous risk factor modification program and was retested a year later. The PET scan demonstrated that he now had major improvements in all three arteries. So this is a good technique for measuring flow reserve and a reminder that we can even reverse narrowed heart arteries if we really work at it with lifestyle changes like diet and exercise and, if needed, with cholesterol-lowering agents.

The PET-CT combination scanning with both rubidium and radioactive glucose allows the radiologist to see areas of the heart that are scarred and not working and compare them to areas that are normal and functional. This is a good test for patients who have had a heart attack and may now have some evidence of developing heart failure. Now the physician can know exactly *where* and *how* damaged the heart muscle is and then make critical decisions about medical therapy, surgery, or both.

Although the older SPECT test is common at most hospitals and gives the needed answer for most situations, it may well be eclipsed by these new techniques with their ability to provide more detailed information on more complex situations. That said, a new test with SPECT, using a radioactive fatty acid abbreviated as BMIPP, has great promise for determining if pain a few hours before represented cardiac blood flow problems. Frequently a patient will come to the ER or his physician saying that he had pain last night or out on the golf course, but it is now gone. The electrocardiogram is normal now because the blood flow has recovered. But a SPECT test using BMIPP will be abnormal if the problem was reduced blood supply to the heart muscle hours before. BMIPP has memory ability of what happened, and this shows up as an abnormal scan result even though the patient feels fine now. This could prove to be a valuable test in the coming years.

Molecular Imaging—Putting It All Together

With molecular imaging your doctor will be better able to make an early diagnosis of cancer, see what is happening inside atherosclerotic plaques in your coronary arteries, study your arthritic joints, and know if you are in the earliest stages of Alzheimer's disease.

Personalized medicine will come closer to reality as molecular imaging develops during the next five to fifteen years. For example, a person's cancer can be biopsied, cells placed in a mouse, and the tumor allowed to grow. Now use an agent that will bind to the tumor cells and inject it into the mouse. It will bind to the tumor and show it on an imaging device, such as PET, MRI, or optical. Next, treat the mouse with a drug or biologic expected to be effective for this type of tumor. Or use a new experimental drug that has not been tested much in humans yet. Immediately scan the mouse to see if the drug has been taken up by the tumor cells. Then scan again in hours or days to see if the drug has had the desired effect of killing the tumor cells.

All this can be done in the mouse today, and the results can be observed with various imaging devices. Soon these techniques can become commonplace for human use, and as a result the physician can feel reasonably confident that the drug or biologic agent will indeed work in the patient. Personalized medicine, again.

MAMMOGRAPHY—ANATOMY NOW, BUT MOLECULAR INFORMATION IN A FEW YEARS

Mammograms are done by X-ray, and every woman knows that around age forty, she should have a mammogram done regularly. Deaths from breast cancer are down mostly because cancers are being found earlier—when they are smaller, more treatable, and less likely to have spread outside the breast. Mammography is quite good for detecting tumors in postmenopausal women, but is much less sensitive for premenopausal women. It is only about 40 percent sensitive in younger women, meaning that when something is found on mammography and then one looks back to last year's mammogram, it was in fact there, but not sufficiently obvious to raise an alarm. If the radiologist sees *micro calcifications,* this leads to a high level of suspicion. But only about 50 percent of small breast cancers have micro calcifications, so the others tend to be missed. This is an area that needs improvement.

Digital mammography is one new approach with a couple of advantages. One is that it allows screening at a distance. A woman can be screened in her own community and the image sent to a central location where an expert radiographer can read it. This can reduce travel time for patients, but it also reduces the one-on-one personal interaction value that can also help to allay concerns and fears. It also means that a difficult image can be sent electronically to a major center for review by an expert who specializes in mammography.

Digital radiography has another advantage in that it can give higher contrast resolution and this will show micro calcifications better than routine mammography. Finally, since the image is digital, it can be manipulated in the computer by the radiologist. This allows for more detailed analysis, which in the past could only be done by having the woman come back for a repeat image—and suffering the anxiety that entails until the repeat image is completed and read.

Unlike X-ray mammography, MRI mammography is almost 100 percent sensitive at any age. Its downside is that it is not terribly specific; it will pick up nonmalignant conditions as though they might be cancer, especially in women who have fibrocystic changes of their breasts. For MRI to be useful, it needs to be done in conjunction with an injection of gadolinium. This increases the contrast and hence the chance to pick up a lesion.

If you recall our earlier discussion about the compound choline, elevated in many cancer cells, then you will appreciate that a way to increase specificity in MRI is to use MRI spectroscopy to look for areas with higher choline concentrations—these will be elevated in cancer, but not in fibrocystic changes. Given these attributes, there is a good possibility that MRI, although it requires an injection and takes longer to do, may become the screening technique of choice for high-risk younger women. This might include women who have a strong family history of breast cancer, a known genetic mutation like BCRA-1 or 2, or those with a prior lumpectomy who need follow-up.

But X-ray mammography is still the standard approach. One method to improve detection is *computer-aided detection* (CAD). This is being rapidly adopted and is based on a computer software algorithm that screens the image and literally marks suspicious areas for the radiologist to look at. The same type of methodology is now beginning to be used in lung screening with CAT images.

Routine mammography is not perfect, but it has proven valuable in detecting small cancers. As a result, deaths from breast cancer have fallen dramatically in recent years. The better news is that new mammography technologies being developed will be even more accurate and effective in the coming years.

INTERVENTIONAL RADIOLOGY

We tend to think of radiology as used for making diagnoses. But it is increasingly being used for treatment, hence the term *interventional.*

A cardiac catheterization with angioplasty to open an artery and placement of a stent to hold it open is *interventional radiology.* Now surgeons and radiologists working together can fix aortic aneurysms in the abdomen without open surgery. And they can insert those tiny platinum coils in the brain aneurysm and effectively cure it without open neurosurgery. The person with a bleeding liver from trauma can have the bleeding stopped with a catheter insertion via the groin artery, rather than with surgery. I will discuss this in more detail in the chapter on the operating room, but suffice to say here that this is a true megatrend—another of those transformational technologies in medicine that is rapidly advancing.

Interventional Radiology

- Repair Aortic Aneurysms
- Repair Brain Aneurysms
- Destroy Tumors in Liver, Lung
- Stop Bleeding in Liver, Intestine, Spleen
- Open Artery to Kidney Causing High Blood Pressure
- Insert Stents/Balloon Angioplasty
- Many Others

IMAGING ELSEWHERE THAN IN THE RADIOLOGY DEPARTMENT

We are accustomed to thinking of radiology as done in the radiology department of a hospital or in a special radiology suite in an outpatient facility. But that is changing—and rather rapidly. For example, a good emergency room will have a fast CT scanner and a handheld ultrasound. A trauma center will have a fast CT scanner, perhaps one of the special scanners that can scan the whole body in just a few seconds, and it will also have ultrasound. Cancer centers will have mammography and the specialized breast imaging techniques, such as MRI and the ability to do stereoscopic breast biopsies. In the operating room, we will find intraoperative MRI, intraoperative ultrasound, intraoperative X-rays, and the neuronavigational devices that are discussed in chapter six.

What we are seeing in radiology is a real transformation to imaging, since X-rays are only one of the modalities used. And we are seeing multiple medical disciplines coming together like never before to solve problems. Think of the engineers and computer specialists who have created the CAT scanners. The nuclear medicine experts, the radiographers, the molecular biologists, and even the nano experts who are working on ways to use PET and other scanners to detect disease both anatomically and functionally, and then to monitor treatment. This is perhaps the ultimate megatrend, having disparate fields come together to solve a problem akin to the "man to the moon" program of the 1960s. Hopefully, the new technologies will be designed and defined to relate directly to the individual's problem with more and more personalized medicine.

To repeat an example, take a tumor sample from a patient, place it in a mouse where it can grow, treat it with the drug proposed for the patient, and scan it. Determine if the drug or agent kills the tumor cells in the mouse as measured immediately with the small animal scanner. Then with that information, go back to the patient with an individualized treatment—and monitor the patient's tumor and its treatment with one of the new molecular scanners. This personalized medicine scenario will play out in many situations in the not-too-distant future.

MEGATRENDS IN IMAGING

Four megatrends have emerged in imaging. First, it is possible to obtain exquisite anatomic images of the body from the outside with no pain or fuss. These truly incredible pictures are exceptionally valuable in making a diagnosis or in telling a surgeon in advance what to expect. To some degree this is an evolutionary advancing process, getting better each year with greater resolution and greater speed. But at some point the megatrend becomes truly disruptive or transformational. Such is the case when you can now visualize the coronary arteries with CT scans and avoid catheterization, detect lung cancer early enough to cure it in most patients, or do a virtual colonoscopy.

The second megatrend is that imaging devices can now detect function and even detect molecular changes and actions in cells—and describe these molecular activities as pictures. So we can see how a tumor is taking up sugar or how much blood is flowing through each coronary artery or how the inflammatory cells in the carotid artery plaque are behaving—and how this has changed over time. Here again, these will become transformational changes, uniquely making it possible to understand the functions of the body in a noninvasive manner, such as studying a patient's tumor response to a drug and making the appropriate decisions as a result.

THE MEGATRENDS

■ Incredibly Detailed Anatomic Images

■ Functional/Molecular Analysis of Organs and Cells Via Images

■ Interventional Radiology Replacing Surgery

■ All Digitized

— Manipulate into virtual procedures

— Easy to keep your own data

These new techniques make it increasingly possible to do procedures less invasively than standard surgery and do them outside of the operating room, using *interventional radiology* (discussed in detail in chapter 6). Finally, because all of the images are now being obtained digitally, they can be manipulated to create virtual colonoscopies and the like. They can be studied in numerous ways such as examining the anatomy before surgery—no surprises. And you can have a copy of your images to save for future comparisons. There is a great convergence of imaging with many types of therapy. It is new, and it is a true disruptive technology. Medicine will never be the same. These are the trends and although we have reviewed what is happening, you can be sure that the pace of innovation will only quicken during the next five to fifteen years.

WHAT YOU SHOULD KNOW

Today we can see inside the body to a degree unexpected just a few years ago. This will accelerate dramatically in coming years and will be particularly important in preparing for an operation, for the early and rapid diagnosis of the cause of chest pain, and for the rapid diagnosis of subtle abdominal pain. We will increasingly be able to visualize function rather than just anatomy, particularly of the brain, heart, and vessels, and we'll compare cancerous tissue to normal tissues. Developing technologies will allow us to concurrently obtain and then fuse anatomical images with functional images as can be done with a combination of PET and CT scanning or with functional MRI and MRI spectroscopy.

Increasingly, small instruments such as the ultrasound or the endoscopic video capsule capture information. We are not only improving diagnosis but also monitoring treatment. We are going to learn more and more about the normal function of the brain with techniques like functional MRI and PET to see what happens during meditation, during empathy, and during pain. The result is that in the coming years the accuracy of diagnosis will continue to advance, as will improvements in the delivery of care and the follow-up to that care. It means much more personalized medicine—medicine designed for the individual.

WHAT YOU CAN DO

My suggestion is that you become aware of these technologies, at least in a general way, so that you can ask your doctor questions before being sent for an imaging study. Certainly you will want to ask what it is that the doctor wants to learn. And what does your physician feel is the best technique to learn what needs to be learned about you and what is inside of you? Once you have that information, then the question is: What radiology site or practice has the best equipment for the specific test? And most important, which radiographers have the most experience?

None of us know when we are going to have a heart attack or a stroke. But just as you may have planned with your family what to do in case of a fire, such as what window to go out and where to meet outside, you might want to have plans in case you or a family member should develop chest pain or evidence of a stroke. If you or a loved one were having chest pain, do you know which emergency rooms have the new multislice scanners that would be best for evaluating your heart in rapid order? If you or a loved one were having signs that suggested a stroke, would you know where to be taken—and fast—to get appropriately scanned so that tPA, if appropriate, could be given immediately or so that those tiny platinum coils could be inserted to eliminate a brain aneurysm and bleeding into the brain?

Heavy-duty questions and ones most of us have not taken the time and energy to research in advance. Meanwhile, consider that these advances in imaging will allow your physician to offer you medical care designed just for you—one more instance of personalized medicine—and, hopefully, personalized in a way that "rehumanizes" health care—for you.

CHAPTER 5

Devices—Small and Powerful

Engineering advances and the ability to put enormous information algorithms onto semiconductors have created rapid, remarkable progress in devices for medical use. I will review just a few of the recently introduced devices—chosen no more scientifically than because I found them interesting and illustrative of what is being developed—and try to predict what types of devices may be coming down the pike. Many of these devices allow doctors to improve body function with relatively minimally invasive procedures and technologies. Some are a good follow-up to our discussion of interventional radiology. The discussion is divided into sections: **cardiac-related devices** (devices for stimulating the heart, devices for unclogging arteries, cardiac assist devices, and devices used in heart surgery); **brain-related devices** (devices that stimulate the brain for epilepsy, depression, Parkinson's, and other problems); **combined diagnostic and treatment device** (ultrasound); **nanodevices** (devices smaller than can be seen with a microscope); and **biomaterials** (cellular tissue engineering). Let's look first at devices that can benefit those with heart problems.

CARDIAC-RELATED DEVICES

Pacemakers, Defibrillators, and Electrophysiology

Cardiac pacemakers have been available for thirty to forty years.

The original ones were close to the size of a pack of cigarettes. The device had a battery and a mechanism to send an electrical stimulation via a wire to a portion of the heart. Usually a pacemaker is inserted under the skin on the chest, just below the collarbone on the left side. Then the wire from the pacemaker is advanced through a vein into the right side of the heart. There it is positioned to touch the lining cells of the heart.

The electrical stimulation from the pacemaker along the wire directs the heart to beat, but the amount of electrical charge is minimal enough that the patient cannot feel it. The original pacemakers, by today's standards, were rather simplistic and the battery needed to be charged frequently. They were capable of being set for a single heart rate, say seventy-two beats per minute. This was a big advance and even lifesaving, but when you are sleeping, you do not need a heart rate of seventy-two, and when you are trying to carry two bags of groceries up the stairs, you need a much faster heart rate.

Today, a pacemaker is about the size of a book of matches, with a long battery life and powerful capabilities. It can be set to have the heart beat at any given rate, but it can also detect when the body needs to increase or decrease that rate. In short, it can sense the needs of the patient. The device can pick up the heart's own electrical activity and make a decision to override it if the heart is beating with an abnormal rhythm, such as one called *paroxysmal atrial tachycardia* (PAT).

But sometimes a minimally invasive procedure can permanently eradicate the problem. A patient of mine, the head chef at an excellent restaurant, would develop PAT intermittently, but usually at very inopportune times. Once he was driving his car on Interstate-95 and literally had to pull off on the side of the road because his heart rate climbed to 220 beats per minute making him dizzy and foggy-headed. Another time he was preparing dinners and had to stop and lie down because of the PAT. Sometimes it would stop on its own, but frequently he had to rush to the nearest emergency room where he would be given an injection of a drug that would break this abnormal rhythm and bring his heart rate back to normal.

When a new procedure called *cardiac electrophysiology* first became available, he volunteered to have it. In that procedure, a catheter is inserted in the groin and advanced up to the heart. The cardiologist checks all areas of the atria (the upper chambers of the heart) to find the area of the heart that was putting out this abnormal rhythm. Once this "over-excitable" region was found, the area was cauterized; essentially the cells in that area were destroyed so that they could no longer create this abnormal rhythm. He has been just fine since.

Electrophysiology (EP) has other uses as well. Atrial fibrillation is a good example of EP being used in a newly developed fashion. It is an "irregularly irregular" heartbeat, originating in a portion of the heart called the left atrium or the nearby pulmonary veins. Usually thought of as occurring in individuals with problems in their mitral heart valve that cause the left atrium to swell, it can occur in perfectly heart-healthy individuals—and be a real nuisance, causing light-headedness, palpitations in the chest, and an inability to carry out some normal activities.

The incidence of atrial fibrillation—whether from disease or in normal hearts—increases with advancing age. Electrophysiology can map out where atrial fibrillation begins, usually in the veins emptying from the lungs into the left atrium of the heart. So using the same ablation or cauterization process, the area where the fibrillation starts can be isolated to prevent it from causing this increasingly frequent problem for older individuals. The procedure can take many hours, because instead of treating just one spot, the catheter must treat a ring or circle around the area to block the electrical activity there from entering the rest of the heart. But it is still a less-invasive procedure than surgery, for example, and it usually works for those without underlying heart disease.

Returning to the pacemaker, it can be used to control some heart irregularities like PAT. The pacemaker can override the abnormal rhythm and get the heart rate down to a normal speed. I think the real point about pacemakers is that they have made the quality of life much better for many and indeed have saved many lives over the years. The advances in pacemakers are moving along rapidly, with the ability to engineer smaller sizes, with longer-lasting batteries and, with the ability to pack more complex software circuits into the chips on board.

A new use of pacemakers is to improve circumstances for patients with heart failure. More and more people who have heart attacks are surviving only to go home to find some degree of heart damage has occurred, such that their heart can no longer pump at a normal level. Picture this: The heart fills up with blood and then squeezes it out with each beat. But in heart failure the heart just cannot squeeze well enough, and as a result only a much smaller proportion of blood (the *ejection fraction*) is actually expressed from the heart out into the aorta and conveyed to the body. It is now possible to take a pacemaker and instead of having one wire (called a *lead*) go into the heart, multiple leads can go to different areas. If just one lead were to stimulate the heart, then the contraction would start at that spot and then, as the electrical activity spread, eventually contract the rest of the heart. But normally the heart contracts in a synchronous motion.

So by having multiple leads going to multiple sites in the heart, it is possible to make the heart contract in a much more efficient manner. For people with heart failure, this improvement in efficiency can make the difference between being unable to engage in many of life's normal activities and having a much better quality of life. Perhaps they cannot run the marathon, but it can make the difference between being able to walk only a few steps and being able to take the dog around the block.

All of these advances came about as the integrated circuit on semiconductors advanced, the software developed, the size decreased, and battery life improved dramatically. The onboard computer allows for adjustment of rate and rhythm on demand so that the fairly simple pacemakers of yesterday have become very complex and sophisticated. And they will continue to do so. Closely related to pacemakers, and developed out of the same technology, are cardioverters/defibrillators.

These devices are implanted in the same way and can monitor the heart's electrical activity. Initially, they had to be implanted in the operating room; now they are placed in the electrophysiology laboratory. The monitoring device can tell if the heart is beating in an abnormal manner that is, or may soon develop into, a life-threatening situation. But let's step back for a minute. When an individual has a heart attack, the initial risk is that the lack of blood flow to an area of the heart will "irritate" those cells resulting in abnormal electrical activity. One of the major risks that occurs early while a heart attack is developing is not only an irregularity of the heart's normal rhythm, but also a beat that is either so fast it progresses to useless electrical activity called *ventricular fibrillation* or sometimes to total electrical stoppage. In either case, no blood is being pumped by the heart and immediate death follows.

This is why we have all learned that at the first evidence of chest pain it is critical to call 911. The emergency medical technicians (EMTs) are trained to monitor the heart while en route to the hospital and to use a defibrillator if necessary, should the heart rhythm degenerate into ventricular fibrillation or total electrical stoppage. Indeed, this quick response by EMTs at home or in the ambulance or by health care providers in hospitals deserves major credit for reducing deaths from heart attacks.

It is well known that a person who has had one cardiac arrest is much more likely to have a second one. So for this reason, implantable defibrillators have been placed with the idea that, should ventricular fibrillation occur again, the device will detect it and shock the heart internally to bring it back to its normal rhythm. This ability for the device to recognize the early evidence of impending heart stoppage due to electrical imbalance and to correct it has saved many thousands of lives.

You may have read that a few devices have malfunctioned, resulting in ventricular fibrillation that the defibrillator did not stop. The manufacturing companies are working to correct these internal software problems. In the meantime it is important to remember that, notwithstanding the deaths of a few individuals, these devices have saved the lives of countless numbers who otherwise would have died.

Angioplasty and Stents

Heart attacks are caused by the partial or total blockage of one or more of the arteries going to the heart *(coronary arteries)*. Without blood flow, oxygen can't get to the muscle cells. First, these cells are injured, which causes pain, and then if the blood flow remains low, the cells of the heart muscle die. Once that happens, that part of the heart muscle cannot properly pump blood. Cardiac surgeons can fix this problem by using a vein from the leg to fashion a bypass around the blockage, an operation called *coronary artery bypass grafting* (CABG). This approach has been effective and indeed lifesaving.

For the past fifteen years or so, balloon angioplasty has provided a less-invasive, valuable approach. Here is how it works. A catheter is inserted in the large artery in the groin (or occasionally the arm) and is snaked up to the heart. It is then turned to enter the coronary arteries, dye is injected, X-rays are taken, and the blockages in the various arteries are evaluated. Then the catheter is advanced to the area of the blockage and actually passed through the blocked area.

The next step is to blow up a "balloon," which surrounds the last few inches of the catheter. This literally squeezes the blockage out of the artery. The balloon is deflated, and the catheter is pulled back a bit, and dye is once again injected. Now the X-rays will show if the artery has been opened. Balloon angiography is quite effective, has relatively few side effects, and is certainly easier on the patient than having open-heart surgery. The biggest problem has been that the artery may start to clog up again, which is called *restenosis*.

Engineers working with cardiologists developed something called *stents*. These are metal scaffolds that when in place will force the artery to remain open. But there are spaces between the metal wires of the stent, and cells can grow through and back into the artery. While a stent is much better at preventing restenosis, a substantial number of stented arteries do begin to close up again.

Let me tell you the story of Robert Packer. He is a hard-driving businessman and was the CEO of a large and successful manufacturing business. He was a little overweight, had slightly increased blood pressure, and had adult-onset diabetes, although it was relatively mild. He exercised only occasionally. He worked long hours. But the process used in his company was eclipsed by a competitor's new process, and his firm began to rapidly lose business.

It was clear that Mr. Packer had tried to deal with the issue as soon as it came to his attention. But it cost the company seriously in terms of money, prestige, business, and stock value. Ultimately, the board of directors decided that, while it was obviously not Mr. Packer's direct fault, it was best for the company to have new leadership. Once a man with essentially no free time, he suddenly had all day, every day to think about what went wrong, how he might have averted the problem, and what he might do next.

His blood pressure started to rise, his blood sugar became harder to control, and his weight went up a bit more. Soon he was in the emergency room complaining of chest pain. The cardiac catheterization laboratory found an obstruction of one of his coronary arteries and performed an angioplasty. Three months later, he was back and repeat catheterization showed that the artery was once again partially occluded. This time, he had not only the angioplasty but also the placement of a stent.

Three more months went by, and he was back in the emergency room again with pain in the chest. Now an angiogram showed that another coronary artery was developing a blockage, and once again he had an angioplasty and the introduction of a stent. Not long after that, he was offered a new job. It was not at the same level as before, but it was a real job with real work and good pay. It also got him into an office setting every day, interacting with other individuals. His blood pressure started to come down, his blood sugar came under control, he started an organized program of weight loss and exercise, and he has had no more chest pain.

What Mr. Packer needed was some purpose in his life and to get past his hurt and anger, but along the way, he needed three angioplasties and two stents to help keep his coronary arteries functioning.

Coronary Artery Stent

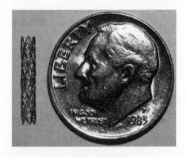

Courtesy Thomas Jemski, University of Maryland School of Medicine.

Stents have had a significant impact on maintaining the patency of angioplasty procedures. Cells still do grow through those stents, however, so the next generation of stents, which have been available for only about three years, has a drug fused to the stent wall. These drugs slowly diffuse from the metal structure, therefore are called *drug-eluting stents,* and they prevent the cells of the walls of the arteries from recreating the obstruction.

These stents are considerably more expensive but they seem to be much better at preventing restenosis and, hence, reduce the need to return to the cath lab or for coronary artery bypass graft surgery. So the increased costs would seem to be balanced by fewer costs from repeat procedures or surgery. But there is concern that they are associated with thrombosis (blood clots) that can lead to new obstructions. Of course, the drug-eluting stents are patented, and that will tend to keep the price up for a while, but perhaps as new approaches become available, competition will cause prices to fall.

A new technology being studied is a resorable stent, which will be put in place like a standard metal stent but after some months will be totally reabsorbed by the body. These types of stents, some made with a magnesium base and others with a polymer base, will overcome the difficulty current stents pose when there is need for rework in the same area. The stent is still there and nearly impossible to remove without open surgery. The absorbable stent might be useful for children who need repeated interventions, young children whose vessels are growing, and older patients who need repeated procedures. So far, the results have been mixed in that the stents work fine initially and are absorbed, but the vessel frequently has restenosis.

Another approach for angioplasty is using a balloon that is coated with a drug that comes off during the procedure, diffusing into the cells of the vessel wall to prevent the cells from growing back. This means a stent will not be needed and there will be less restenosis. If these work out, it could be a major advance.

Finally, be aware that new approaches with lasers are being studied to open clogged coronary arteries and arteries with long blockages such as those in the leg. And in a process called *atherectomy* mechanical devices can actually enter the coronary or peripheral artery and cut and remove the plaque. If done before an angioplasty, this means that there is less debris to squeeze back into the vessel wall.

Cardiac Assist Devices

Let's consider some other devices that can be helpful for patients with heart problems, in particular, patients with heart failure. I will illustrate with the story of Ron Caspian, a fifty-nine-year-old analyst with one of the think tanks that surround Washington, DC. In the fall of 2002, he developed some chest discomfort one Saturday morning. He drove himself to the nearby emergency room where it was quickly confirmed that he was having a heart attack.

Indeed, his heart rapidly began to fail, and he was rushed to the cardiac catheterization laboratory where an angioplasty was performed. This opened up the major blocked artery, but his heart muscle was dangerously weak. His cardiologist telephoned a cardiac surgeon at the hospital where I worked and asked if he could transfer the patient while adding, "But I'm not sure you'll be willing to accept him."

The surgeon, never one to give up easily, asked, "Why not?"

"Well, because despite the angioplasty, his pulse is very rapid, his blood pressure is zip, his kidneys are not making much urine, and his blood flow is so limited he is semi-comatose."

"Send him quick," said the surgeon, who geared up to insert a cardiac assist device. The idea is to let the heart rest while a mechanical device does much of the pumping for the heart. It is hoped that after a few days the heart may regain some of its function and be able to carry on its role once again.

So Mr. Caspian was transferred, and the cardiac assist device was installed. It is about the size of a fist and fits around a portion of the heart; through a pneumatic system it helps the heart pump blood to the body. The large pneumatic driver that powers the assist device is housed in a small suitcaselike affair that the patient must keep next to him all the time.

I saw this gentleman when I came to work on Monday morning, and he certainly did not look well—although the surgeon was quite pleased. By Wednesday, Mr. Caspian was sitting up and really looking pretty good. This was remarkable because there is no question he would have died on Saturday afternoon if not for the quick work of the cardiologist by doing an emergency angioplasty and the cardiac surgeon by implanting the cardiac assist device. After a few more days, however, it became evident that Mr. Caspian's heart was just not going to recoup and that he would need a heart transplant to survive. But a heart for transplantation rarely becomes available; in fact, most patients die before a heart is ever available.

What to do? The cardiac surgeon decided—with the advice and consent of both the patient and his wife—to try a new device. It is about the size of a D battery, like the one you use in your flashlight, with a little electric turbine inside; yet it can move blood, not quite in the amounts that a normal heart can pump, but still enough to keep the body functioning at a fair level of activity.

The surgeons tell me it is quite easy—for a skilled surgeon—to insert, but the description I am about to give you may not sound all that simple. First, the chest is opened, and then the tip end (apex) of the heart is opened, and this battery-sized device is inserted and sewn into place. Coming out from the heart is a tube about an inch in diameter, which goes to the aorta, that large artery that sends blood to the rest of the body. A wire from the little turbine comes out through the chest and hooks onto a battery about the size of a cell phone that can be hooked to your belt. The chest is then sewn up. Using electricity from the battery, the turbine moves the blood from the heart out through the tube up to the aorta and into the body.

This device is much smaller than the larger assist device that Mr. Caspian first had installed; it can be left in place for quite some time, and it runs on batteries. Indeed, some even think that this may prove to be a long-term alternative to a heart transplant, a "destination" device if you will. This was placed into Mr. Caspian's chest, and he did great. He was soon up and about and after a time went home.

Then about three months later, a heart became available and he had a cardiac transplant. I saw him one day in the hospital coffee shop, and he said that he was going to retire. "I've been eligible for three years now and frequently thought about it, but after 9/11 there was so much work to be done at our organization that I just couldn't leave. But now I know I need to avoid the stress and take care of myself. I have a new lease on life, and I want to make good use of it."

That all sounded pretty logical to me, but when I saw him again six months later he said, "Well, I just started back to work. They made me an offer I couldn't refuse. I really need to get out of the house and do some constructive things. But I will be careful. I feel really good, but I do know I need to not get overstressed."

There is much work in progress to find a way to prevent the body from rejecting transplanted organs. It is proving to be very complicated. When you modify one part of the immune mechanism with a drug, then other systems are affected as well. But there is real progress and immune tolerance will become a reality in the next five to fifteen years. This will mean that organs will not be rejected acutely or over time, powerful drugs with serious long-term side effects will not be needed anymore, and an organ from a donor may be able to be used for any person, not just one with a closely related tissue type.

Some day in the near future, we will not have to worry about finding a human donor. Scientists are hard at work trying to genetically modify animals so that their organs can be used and not be rejected by the human body. This is called *xenotransplantation*. I do not know if hearts from an animal, such as a pig, will be ready for human transplantation in the next five years, but I suspect that they will be within the next fifteen years. This will solve the donor issue and mean that a heart transplant can be an option much earlier in the course of heart failure, unlike today where it is reserved for those who are exceptionally ill and near death. Xenotransplantation would work for other organs as well, such as kidneys and livers.

Devices Used in Heart Surgery

Let's consider some other approaches to the treatment of various heart diseases. When a coronary artery bypass graft surgery is done (CABG) the patient is placed on the heart-lung machine. This is one of the greatest devices developed during the mid-twentieth century because it allows the surgeon to actually stop the heart so it will not beat during the bypass of the coronary arteries or the repair of congenital defects or damaged valves. It works—and it works well—but complications include bleeding and mental changes can occur after the procedure.

A number of approaches have been developed to allow the surgeon to work on the heart while it is still beating—"off pump" CAGB procedures. One device is called an *octopus* because it has a series of small suction cups that hold a portion of the heart steady while the surgeon works there, while allowing the rest of the heart to continue to beat and pump blood. Originally about 20 percent of patients were eligible for this type of off pump bypass surgery, but some surgeons find that they can do 50 to 70-plus percent of patients using this technology.

The grafts implanted in this fashion, however, may not remain open as long after the procedure as do the veins put in patients whose hearts have been stopped to place them on the heart-lung machine. But certainly for patients who are at greater risk for pump problems, such as those with diseased aortas, severe pulmonary disease, liver disease, or some type of bleeding problem, the off-pump procedure becomes a real boon. A thought to consider: If you or a loved one needs cardiac surgery and are told that it will be done without the heart-lung machine, then you want to be absolutely certain that the surgeon doing the procedure is highly skilled and does this frequently.

Another new approach is the method for "harvesting" the vein in the legs for the bypass graft. Traditionally, the surgeon or assistant would make a long incision the length of the leg and remove the saphenous vein. This could be divided up for the various grafts used to bypass the blocked coronary arteries. Obviously, this incision was painful, could get infected, and was aesthetically unpleasant for the patient. So a device was developed that allows the vein to be removed from the inside. A very small incision is made high on the leg, and the device is inserted into the vein and then "pulls" it out without the need for that long incision. The vein segments are just as good, and patients certainly prefer this approach.

Here is another device that would have seemed impossible just a few years ago. I learned that a colleague that I had not seen for some years had had a stroke, so I telephoned to see how he was doing. His wife told me that he had been at an event and felt dizzy and a little confused at the end. He was seen by neurologists who diagnosed a mini stroke. The episode recurred a month later, and they then noticed that he had a *patent foramen ovale* in his heart.

Basically, this is a normal opening between the two sides of the heart during fetal development, but it closes up in most people near the time of birth— but not in everyone. He was one of those individuals. Apparently he had had a blood clot in his leg, and a piece broke off (an *embolus*), traveled up to the right side of his heart, and then passed across the foramen ovale into the left side of his heart. From there, it could travel up the *carotid arteries* (the big arteries that go up the neck to the brain) and lodge in his brain.

Only a few years ago, it would have taken open-heart surgery and the heart-lung machine to repair the abnormality. But his procedure was much simpler and much safer. Using a catheter in the manner we have previously discussed, the cardiologist found the opening. From there he was able to place a patch over the hole in such a way that it was set on the side of the heart where the pressure is higher, thus holding it in place. With time, the heart's normal cells will start to grow over it, and it will become an integral part of the divider of the right and left side of his heart. No longer can blood clots pass across, so he cannot have this type of embolic stroke again. That is great news, but equally great is the fairly noninvasive approach. It only took an hour or so to complete in the cardiac catheterization laboratory, instead of in the cardiac surgical operating room.

BRAIN-RELATED DEVICES

Brain Stimulation

A device that looks a lot like a pacemaker can be used to reduce the frequency of epileptic seizures. Epilepsy is quite common. Various drugs can

help and may totally prevent seizures, or at least reduce their frequency substantially. But some individuals are not adequately treated with drugs alone.
Cindy Matheson was such an individual.

She had been having seizures since early childhood. She was bright, ener-
getic, and enthusiastic, but as the seizures became more common and frequent, the medications had to be increased. This made her drowsy, so in high
school it became increasingly difficult to study. She started college but found
that she could not study well enough, so she began reducing the dose of her
drugs. She promptly started having seizures again.

Every time she increased the dosage back to what she was supposed to
take, she could not study effectively, yet when she reduced the dosage she had
more and more seizures. This was certainly a catch-22. She was anxious to
complete her college education, but it looked as if it would be impossible.

Then came a new approach. Her doctor took a device that looks much like
a pacemaker, implanted it under the skin below the collarbone, and tunneled
the lead not to the heart, but to where the vagus nerve travels through the
neck on the left side. The vagus nerve comes from the brain down through
the neck and into the chest and abdomen, where it helps to control heart
rate, digestion, and other important functions in our body. It is part of the
parasympathetic nervous system.

The wire from the implanted device is attached to the vagus nerve, and
the nerve can now be stimulated with low-intensity electric pulses. Remarkably
this has been found to reduce the frequency of seizures for many individuals.
Some are even seizure-free while others can reduce their drug dosages—a major
improvement in quality of life, as it certainly was for this young college student.

Here is another use of vagal nerve stimulation. A year ago a gentleman
called to say that his wife was suffering from fairly serious depression. They
were not satisfied with her medical care and asked if I could recommend a
psychiatrist in their area. I checked with some colleagues and called back with
a name. The next I heard was about six months later when my acquaintance
called back to say that his wife and he were both very pleased with the psychiatrist, but that she was still having substantial difficulty with depression.

She had been on multiple and various medications, but they really had
not done the job. So their psychiatrist suggested they consider a new and still
investigational approach to treatment, which was vagal nerve stimulation. I
knew about vagal nerve stimulation for epilepsy, but I was not aware of its use
for depression. So I called a neurosurgeon that I knew put in these devices for
epilepsy and asked what he had heard.

To my surprise, he had just finished installing about twenty as part of a national study. He directed me to a psychiatrist who was the lead investigator. I learned that this is certainly not a panacea, but it does seem to work for some people with intractable depression. The outside of the vagus nerve has the fibers that go to the brain; the inside of the nerve has the fibers that come from the brain to the various organs in the body. The leads (wires) from the device are attached to the outside edges of the nerve, and the nerve is stimulated. Apparently, the impulses go up to the brain but not down to the organs. Many people have shown remarkable improvement.

I reported all of this back to my acquaintance and gave him the name of the lead investigator. At the time I am writing this paragraph, his wife is preparing to have this device inserted. Time will tell how helpful it may be for her.

If you can stimulate the brain from the outside, what about stimulation directly to the inside? Deep brain stimulation uses an electrode placed deep within certain centers of the brain and works something like a brain pacemaker to treat patients with various movement disorders like Parkinson's disease, essential tremors, and dystonia. Patients with these types of disorders get severe tremors, muscle contractions, rigidity, and loss of balance. Even when mild, it can have a substantial effect on the quality of life, and when severe, it can be completely debilitating.

The pacemaker-like device sends a mild electrical stimulation into the deep centers of the brain, where it blocks the impulses that cause the tremors. It is battery-operated with a long life and improves not only a patient's sense of his general health, but his physical functions as well. It is not a cure, but at the same time, it certainly does improve the quality of life for carefully selected individuals. Try to imagine how much better your quality of life would seem if once again you could drink a cup of tea without spilling it.

Deep brain stimulation (DBS) has been used the most in Parkinson's disease so far and is having a real benefit for carefully selected patients. But it is being used more and more for those with tremors. Until now there was no treatment. People with severe hand tremors find they cannot write, have difficulty dressing, and trouble with other ordinary routines of life. DBS usually does not totally rid one of the tremors, but often reduces them.

Dystonia, especially in children and adolescents, can be very disfiguring and disabling with horribly contorted postures. DBS has been having some good successes with that, also. During the next five years, expect to see DBS used for depression and for Tourette's syndrome. There are risks, given that it involves placing an electrode deep into the brain, but the risks can be outweighed by the benefit for those with severe and serious problems. Deep brain stimulation will be refined and improved in the years to come, but the real advance—although not for ten or more years—will be from the combination of genomic information and stem cell advances.

Another concept is called *transcranial magnetic stimulation.* This is also being used for patients with depression who have not responded to drugs or electroshock treatment. Unlike electroshock, the therapy does not cause seizures, there is no pain, anesthesia is not needed, nor is implantation needed, as it is with some of the other stimulation techniques we have just discussed. It is easy, noninvasive, and does not hurt. Basically, it is a magnetic coil held near the scalp that creates a magnetic field, which in turn creates a small electrical current inside the brain. It can be used for depression, but it can also be used for various types of dystonia, cerebral palsy, and possibly even schizophrenia. I am not certain how effective it is, but research is continuing, so time will tell.

In other evaluations of magnetic stimulation of the brain, work is being done that suggests that magnetic coils can block the onset of a migraine headache and possibly even break the headache once it has begun. Given the large number of people with migraine headaches and the relative inadequacy of most treatments today, this could be a real boon if it pans out.

Thoughts to Action

Now let's turn things around and have the brain stimulate the machine. The concept is to implant a device in the brain to detect the brain's signals. These signals—our thoughts—are then translated into mechanical action by moving an arm, leg, hand, or a mechanical arm like the mouse on a computer. Some interesting work is going on in this area with monkeys.

Tiny electrodes are implanted in the brains of monkeys and these record the signals of the brain as the monkey performs tasks. The monkeys have been trained to use a joystick with a computer to place a green circle upon a red circle and when they succeed a robotic arm feeds them. Once the signals are decoded by the researchers, they disconnect the wire from the brain to the signal recorder and connect it instead directly to the robotic arm.

After about two weeks, the monkeys learn that they do not have to move their hands or the joystick to have the robotic arm feed them. Instead, they have learned to just think and, as a result, the robot feeds them directly. This is putting thoughts into action. Think of how this type of technology might help a person who has had a spinal cord injury and cannot transmit information from her functioning brain to her potentially functioning muscles in the arm or legs. Consider also the person who has had a traumatic accident or been injured in warfare and now has a prosthetic limb. The time may well come when brain signals can be sent to a robotically manipulated limb so that it will function as a result of those thoughts. But don't expect this to happen too soon—it is all still very experimental.

DIAGNOSTIC AND TREATMENT DEVICES

I wrote about the smaller, portable ultrasound machine in the chapter on imaging, but it is worth returning to again. This relatively inexpensive device is the ideal way to detect an abdominal aortic aneurysm. It is simple, quick, painless and without false positives. This is important because fifteen thousand or more Americans die each year of aortic aneurysms, whereas more than 90 percent will survive if it is detected and repaired.

There is another developing use of ultrasound. Probably 35 percent of women at some time in their lives will have symptoms from uterine fibroids such as bleeding, increased urination, pain with intercourse, or low back pain. The treatment has traditionally been a hysterectomy, in which the uterus is removed surgically through an incision with a few days in the hospital followed by four to six weeks of recuperation at home. Laparoscopic hysterectomy has shortened the time in the hospital and markedly shortened the recuperation time at home to about a week.

But now high intensity focused ultrasound (HIFU) offers a new approach. Basically, it focuses two beams of ultrasound to a single point. Where the beams meet, harmonic vibration releases thermal energy, which can either vaporize or coagulate tissue. So after an MRI maps out the fibroids, the ultrasound is used to focus beams destroying the tissue. No incisions, no OR, no major anesthesia. This approach is effective in about 70 percent of patients and the recuperation period is very quick.

It is possible that this technology will be used in multiple circumstances during the coming years, as more uses are studied. For example, focused ultrasound could be used to stop internal bleeding. The ultrasound could be used to detect the site of the bleeding, and then the two beams could be focused together on that single point to stop the bleeding—again without an open incision in the OR—all done from the outside with sound waves through the skin.

Another potential use in the years to come will be to get drugs into certain areas of the brain. Our brain has a protective mechanism (the blood brain barrier) that keeps compounds other than glucose and a few others from crossing from the blood to the cells of the brain. It is a great safety device to protect the brain from injury. But it also means that many drugs that we would like to get into the brain cannot, such as many anticancer drugs. HIFU could be aimed in such a manner and intensity that it opens up this barrier on a temporary basis and lets a drug pass in—but only to the areas desired. This technique is still a long way off, but the potential is exciting. There are ongoing evaluations of HIFU in treating brain tumors noninvasively, with the first trials having good success. Trials of treating prostate cancer are also underway. Today, the HIFU device needs the MRI to detect the fibroid (or the tumor, or whatever), but in the future it will be the ultrasound device that can both detect a tumor (or fibroid) and then eliminate it with thermal energy. Prediction: focused ultrasound will have a major impact in the coming years. HIFU has the potential to be a disruptive technology, changing the fundamental way certain problems are addressed.

NANODEVICES

The basic unit of measurement in nanoscience is the *nanometer* (one billionth of a meter), which equals the width of one to ten atoms. It is ten thousand times smaller than a strand of human hair or ten thousand times smaller than an ordinary living cell. New science and technology based on the nanometer refers to the ability to manipulate individual atoms and molecules to build machines on a scale of nanometers or to create materials and structures from the bottom up with novel properties. Nanotechnology, according to the National Science Foundation, could change the way almost everything is designed and made, from automobile tires to vaccines to objects not yet imagined.

The concept is to prepare "smart objects" that can invade small spaces and target specific parts of the body. I did not think that nanomedicine represented a megatrend of sufficient magnitude that it deserved its own chapter, but it certainly is fascinating and some interesting things are being developed. Some researchers expect bioengineering and nanoscience to have a profound impact on the way medicine is practiced.

In 2003, President Bush signed the Twenty-First Century Nanotechnology Research and Development Act. The 2005 budget included one billion dollars for a multiagency, National Nanotechnology Initiative (NNI), and I predict that support for nanotechnology is sure to continue to increase in the coming years. The National Institutes of Health has established a "roadmap" to guide its research directions over the coming years and the roadmap includes specific reference to nanomedicine.

What if doctors could search out and destroy the very first cancer cells that would otherwise cause a tumor to develop in the body? What if a broken part of a cell could be removed and replaced with a miniature biological machine? What if pumps the size of molecules could be implanted to deliver lifesaving medicines precisely when and where they are needed?

These scenarios may sound unbelievable but they are the long-term goals of the NIH Roadmap to Nanomedicine Initiative that we anticipate will yield medical benefits as early as ten years from now (see www.nih.gov). Nanomedicine and biotechnology can be integrated and some see this as perhaps the most exciting scientific and economic development opportunity since the creation of the information technology revolution in the Silicon Valley several decades ago. They see the potential for major improvements in health care, the creation of revolutionary new "smart" materials, and the development of a new generation of environmental sensors as real possibilities. They see that this can rapidly improve the ability to sequence the human genome, develop new techniques for characterizing the internal structure of cells, and allow scientists to duplicate the properties of the molecular machines found in living systems.

Let's consider *nanodevices,* defined by the government as 1) smaller than 100 nm (nanometers)—or much smaller than can even be seen with a microscope—with 2) a new function, and 3) an ability to be controlled externally. The concept is that smaller is better and that recent advances in medicine and nanotechnology can converge. Scientists are making nanoparticles that can be controlled, that function in new ways, and that can get to a cell or get inside the correct cell and deliver a payload such as a drug.

In the field of diabetes the great hope has long been to find a form of insulin that can be taken by mouth. Today, the enzymes in our stomachs and intestines break down the insulin before it can be absorbed into our bloodstream. But scientists are trying to fabricate a porous silicone particle that can travel across the intestinal cell wall and deliver insulin instantly to the blood. If this could be done, it would be like finding the Holy Grail of diabetes— oral insulin. The studies so far have demonstrated an increase in insulin transport across the cell wall by a factor of ten. This is not enough, but it does show a proof of principle, which encourages those working in this field.

Here is another example. A *nanotube* can be formed from silicone dioxide or other similar materials. They form naturally in the right setting but then can be designed to carry certain attachments such as drugs, antibodies, or diagnostic devices—or all three of these. A nanotube can be made from a naturally magnetic material such as magnetite, can have drugs placed inside the tubule, and can have a targeting molecule such as a monoclonal antibody placed on the surface of the tubule.

The nanotubules are injected into the bloodstream via a vein and travel through the body until that monoclonal antibody finds the site that it has been directed to, such as a cancerous cell. The tubule now binds tightly to the cancer cell, and because it is magnetic, it can be detected with an MRI. We know where the cancer cell is and that our nanotube is attached to it. And the drug in the tube is in high concentration right at the site of the cancer cell and nowhere else in the body.

This is an example of how medicine can become personalized to the individual patient. In the United States, about 1.4 million cases of cancer are diagnosed per year, and about six hundred thousand people die from it. More than two hundred types of cancer exist, each with multiple subtypes or variants. With nanoparticles, it should be possible to get right to that cancer—improving the diagnosis, imaging, and treatment—all done with one particle that can target that cancer cell but not the normal cell, image the cancer cell, and deliver the drug. At the time of this writing more than six nanoparticles are either already on the market or at the FDA under evaluation for imaging or therapy.

Here are some other approaches to cancer diagnostics. Another type of nanoparticle is a silicone-based nanowire device. It is designed to recognize electrically minute levels of marker proteins that are overexpressed in cancer and which then circulate in the bloodstream. The device can carry a monoclonal antibody to the protein. This means it will link with the protein if it finds it in the bloodstream. This linkage causes a change in electrical conductance, which can be then detected by the nanowire device.

Watch for articles in newspapers or magazines about using it for early detection of prostate specific antigen (PSA) and others. In fact, it may be possible to put multiple monoclonal antibodies on just one device and in so doing use it to look for multiple different cancers all at one time. I mentioned magnetic emitting nanoparticles earlier. Some new techniques have created the ability to detect breast cancer cells in mice when the tumor is just half a millimeter in size—smaller than this letter *o*.

In the field of therapeutics, any number of drugs or monoclonal antibodies can be attached to nanoparticles and be potentially effective. Again, the concept is to get the drug in high concentrations to exactly where it is needed, yet not cause side effects with other cells in the body. This type of approach will mean producing drugs for each type of cancer. This is quite different from today's drug development approach of "one size fits all."

The concept of personalized medicine means that no one drug will be sold in large quantities. Big pharmaceutical companies, however, are always looking for a blockbuster drug—one that can sell for more than a billion dollars per year. Given this inclination, I wonder whether they will show an interest in this personalized medicine approach of individualized medications. If not, then smaller, entrepreneurial companies hopefully will pick up the slack.

This is all very intriguing and exciting but there is also concern about just where all these nanoparticles will go in the body, where they will reside for many years, and what possible long-term side effects they might have. Look for the FDA to be very cautious in assessing the safety of these new technologies.

BIOMATERIALS

Here is another new concept for you. We might call it tissue engineering. The idea is to create the controlled growth of a living cellular tissue over some form of a solid scaffold, which is preferably biodegradable. Cells could be obtained from a biopsy, grown in large number in a bioreactor, placed on the scaffold to grow into a living tissue, and then transplanted back to the patient at the right stage of development. This might be used, for example, to produce a new form of kidney dialysis machine. It will be based on MEMS (micro-electro-mechanical systems) concepts that will create a miniaturized ultrafiltration device, which some believe will surpass the capability of current hemodialysis machines. If it works as predicted, the system will be more physiologic, with fewer side effects and reduced mortality.

About three hundred thousand individuals in this country with end stage renal disease are on dialysis now, and about 20 percent die each year. Many of the side effects are due to the peaks and valleys of blood chemicals that are found between dialysis—these are molecules that affect the body but that a normal kidney keeps in a steady state of concentration in our blood. Dialysis is done only every two to three days, so there are great variations in blood chemicals.

The new concept would use silicone to make nanoparticles, which will be microfabricated and have a slit shape that mimics the natural pores in the kidneys. The end result would be a miniaturized renal tubule assist device

(RAD) that can be used without the need for a pump, because the heart will do the pumping. This device can be either implanted or it could be worn on the patient's belt. It would replace the need for chronic and regular dialysis on a machine.

Here is another use of microscopic scaffolds to help regenerate cells. You know that when key cells in the brain stop working, as in the case of Alzheimer's or Parkinson's disease or even spinal cord injury, not much can be done today to restore the health of these nonfunctioning cells. One hope is that stem cells will help, but that is certainly well into the future. A few of the current studies use nanotechnology to create some innovative scaffolds that can transport molecular signals directly to the ailing cells. Scientists hope to provide a means to regenerate damaged nerve cells or to restore the junctions between the nerve fibers that were lost because of injury.

MEMS therapies should have a big role in medicine of the future. Today, they are still mostly in the trial stages, but look for these devices to deliver drugs, reside in a specific location in the body, and do specialized work there or get to and attach to a specific cell. Think of them as a computer chip with sensors and effectors integrated together. Just as the chip in your car's airbag system can tell if you are in the beginning of a serious accident or just bumped the curb, a MEMS device will have the ability to differentiate its situation.

They are based on biologically active materials, can be microscopic, can seek out their targets with on-board sensors and then begin a defined action. In many ways, they are similar to nanomedicine devices, but different in construction. MEMS will probably have some uses in the next five years or so; nanomedicine is likely a longer time frame.

LARGER DEVICES

Mostly I have described smaller and smaller devices and approaches to improving medical care in this chapter. But on the other end, there are some very large devices that are making a real difference as well. Radiation therapy is a good example. Here the devices are very large and fill entire rooms. The basic concept is that radiation, if given in a large enough dose, will destroy any tumor. The problem has always been to deliver the needed dose to the cancer but not harm adjacent tissue. That is difficult if the tumor is deep inside the body and the radiation must pass through the normal tissues in order to get to it.

Not so long ago, large lead blocks were constructed to shield as much normal tissue as possible. But that limited options since they were large, had to be made for each patient and were only useful for radiation coming from one direction. Now radiation equipment, linear accelerators, have up to 120 built-in movable metal flanges or leaves called *collimators* that can be preprogrammed by computer for the specific patient and position. This allows the radiation to be administered without the need to construct those large lead shields. And it means that, if desired, the radiation can be given from any number of directions. Let's see why this is important.

Imagine a peach with its pit. We want to give the pit a dose of radiation, which we will arbitrarily call 100 units. But we don't want the peach flesh to get anywhere near that dose. So we could aim the beam at the pit from ten different directions, one after the other and give 10 units at each of these positions. The pit gets the full 100 units because all ten directions are focused on the pit but the peach flesh gets only ten units. But to make this work requires some careful calibrations because the pit is not a smooth round ball. It is rough and is of a different shape depending on the angle you are viewing, just like a tumor.

To deal with this problem, the newest radiation machines, just coming onto the market, have a built-in CT scanner. In our example, it would look at the peach and its pit from each of the ten different positions, take ten scans, and then send that information to a simulator. The simulator in turn sends the data to the treatment planning computer where, under the guidance of a radiation oncologist and a physicist, it calculates the correct dose of radiation and alignment of those metal rods that act as shielding for the peach flesh (normal tissue) while letting the radiation hit the pit (or tumor).

Now the radiation machine, called a *linear accelerator*, can be programmed to move in an arc around the peach (patient) and deliver just the right dose to just the pit (tumor) while sparing most of the normal tissue. And a treatment verification system records exactly what was done automatically. To add to the specificity, imagine a tumor in the lung. Today, we ask the patient to hold their breath while the radiation beam is applied. But we know that breathing can move a tumor a few inches. We want to give the tumor the total needed dose of radiation but not harm much normal lung tissue. So the added CT scanner can help here with the ability to time the radiation to map out the tumor at various points in the breathing cycle and then apply the radiation only at a certain moment during the cycle (called *gating*.) These image-guided radiation therapy devices (IGRT) will offer a major advance. But it is extremely expensive, with the equipment costing about $3.8 million and the shielded vault room costing about $1.5 million. But because they can be operated with assistance from the computer, do not need the work of moving in and out the big lead blocks, and because the simulator and treatment planning is also done largely via computer, it is possible to treat more patients per day on each machine, reducing the cost per patient yet greatly enhancing safety. Further, it may be that the standard of having the patient come back every day for multiple weeks can be reduced to fewer visits. This will also mean more patients can be treated per linear accelerator. As these machines become commonplace—and as they are even further advanced with the ability to deliver radiation from multiple angles adjusting for motion—we will see a remarkable improvement not only in treating cancer but in sparing normal tissue.

MEDICAL AND ENGINEERING INTERACTIONS

It is clear that as physicians bring what today seem like insoluble problems to the attention of engineers, computational scientists, and biologists, solutions seem to be found. One can think of a major academic hospital as a "problem-rich environment" and an engineering university as a "solution-rich environment." But physicians are in their hospitals and engineers are in their own setting, and the two rarely meet unless an organization helps them do so.

The Massachusetts General Hospital in Boston and the Massachusetts Institute of Technology (MIT) have developed the Center for Innovative Minimally Invasive Therapy (CIMIT). The concept is to improve patient care through collaboration between engineers and physicians. The idea is that this collaboration will catalyze the development of innovative technologies emphasizing minimally invasive diagnoses and therapy. Unlike most university research programs, CIMIT is not involved in basic research or in traditional technology development. Rather it exposes "solution-rich" technical people to challenging clinical problems, seeking the least invasive, most cost-effective and scalable techniques while pushing the envelope of technology application and technology transfer.

Much of CIMIT's work is what we might call "matchmaking." Through regular meetings and networking, CIMIT seeks to bring the clinicians and the technologists together and also creates connections with industrial collaborators as well. Some of the nanotechnology and biomaterials that I described are the result of CIMIT bringing together physicians who have a problem—like kidney failure and dialysis—with engineers who can help create a solution.

A similar center has been established at Rutgers University in New

Jersey—the Center for Military Biomaterials Research. This is a network of academia, industry, and the military who provide rapid and effective pathways for identification, development, and utilization of biomaterial-based technologies that will target the military's most urgent health care needs, both on and off the battlefield. They are blending new science and new technology of biomaterial-based products with clinical practice needs. Rather than let technology drive the direction of their long-range research, their approach has been to ask what the market (in this case the military) needs to focus on their customer (in this case the soldier). This results-oriented approach, unlike most university-style approaches, determines the best practices available today in the industry and then drives its research ahead from there.

MEGATRENDS IN THE USE OF DEVICES

As long as problems exist, are identified, and made known to the engineers and others who can help create a solution, those solutions will be devised. Since our economic capitalist system encourages entrepreneurship through the patent process, it is easy to assume and predict that device development will continue at an increasingly accelerated pace.

Devices will become smaller, more powerful, and more useful. Devices already have and will continuously change the practice of medicine in ever more profound ways.

THE MEGATRENDS

- Smaller
- More Powerful
- More Useful
- Multiple Functions at Once (Nano Device)
- Rebuild Organs/Tissues (Biomaterials)

WHAT YOU SHOULD KNOW

Devices are being developed so rapidly that it is impossible to be up-to-date on everything that is available for every disease or condition. Probably the important thing to be aware of is that engineers are making smaller and increasingly more powerful devices that can have a very real impact on medicine—on diagnosis, treatment, and maybe even prevention.

WHAT YOU CAN DO

What I suggest you do is watch the news for what is new. Since these devices are often suitable for visual presentations, they are more likely to reach the news than other things we are discussing in this book. Unfortunately, much of what is reported is often hype and often about untested and untried products, so be on your guard. But at least reading and watching will keep you at the forefront of what is happening and what is being developed. Then if you or a loved one develops a disease or a problem, check the Internet to see what new devices may be available to help with that condition.[1]

Of course, you will want to know that any device of interest has been FDA evaluated and approved, and you will certainly want to talk to your physician. You may come armed with knowledge that your physician does not yet have. Remember that a specialist will probably be up-to-date on most of what is developing in his or her field, but a generalist such as an internist or pediatrician is much less likely to know about the newest devices across all fields. So do not be discouraged if your internist looks at you with a skeptical eye and asks, "What are you talking about?"

Also remember that medicine tends to be conservative—physicians want to see strong proof and a good track record before they will suggest something new for their patients—and most of the time, this is good practice to your benefit. But don't be shy about asking and even pushing some if there appears to be a new approach that could be very helpful to you or a loved one.

CHAPTER 6

The Operating Room of the Future— A Room with a New View

U se your imagination. It's the year 2020, and you need surgery; today is the day. You are the sole occupant in a large operating theater. Nurses and doctors are nowhere in sight. The only other humanlike form is that of a robot—faceless, polished, silent. The room itself is bright white, and gleaming steel arms extend over you. Strategically placed video cameras survey your physical being. Your body is prone and motionless; your mind is in a deep sleep as the action unfolds. A "smart" stretcher has been moving you gently along a conveyor-like belt from one predetermined station to another. As the special gurney supports your inert form, machines carefully monitor your vital signs and the deepest levels of biochemical change within your body.

First stop: a short semicircular tunnel. As you pass through it, invisible rays scan every part of your body. Next stop: the sterilization area, which ensures you won't have any chance of developing a postoperative infection. While you're in the sterilization area, a real-time picture of your inner anatomy and your total body molecular functioning is beamed to a control console just outside the operating room. There your surgeon is reviewing the surgery you're about to have, using a simulator and looking at a virtual you, designing the exact surgery that you need based on your internal anatomy and taking into consideration your cellular functioning. Your final stop is a docking station where a robot is poised to take its orders and make its first incision into your body. Your robotic surgery is about to begin. Of course, you are asleep so you haven't seen any of this. You are in the operating room of the future.

Although I've placed the time for this scenario in the year 2020, elements of it are actually here now and they're gaining in force every year. But before we jump so far ahead, it's important that we pause for a moment and consider surgery in an overall context.

It's fair to say that in the future, patients, surgeons, and the OR will be different. First, fewer surgical procedures overall will need to be done because of other advances in medicine that we've talked about elsewhere in this text.

Not only will fewer procedures be performed, and fewer still be done in the operating room, but also the operating room itself will expand its functions. As our opening example suggests, the OR of the future depends upon technologies such as imaging, simulators, and robotic assistance to the surgeon—an OR that I am calling a *room with a new view.*

NEED FOR FEWER SURGICAL PROCEDURES

In the future, far fewer surgical procedures will be performed. To be sure, we will always need surgeons and surgery for traumatic events and other needs. But as medical care progresses and we become better at preventing many of today's illnesses, less surgery will be needed.

Consider duodenal ulcers. For years, surgery was a mainstay of ulcer care. General surgeons could expect that a major part of their practice would be operating on patients with ulcer disease complications. Then came the new antiulcer drugs like Tagamet and Zantac. These cut off the supply of acid to the stomach and with it the pain and inflammation. Not much later, researchers discovered that ulcers are caused by a germ, a bacterium called *Heliobacter pylori,* which could be eradicated with antibiotics. All of a sudden ulcers could be cured and surgery became a rarity.

Consider coronary artery disease, the problem that causes heart attacks. You know that obstructions occur in the big arteries that feed blood to the heart muscle and if they become completely or near completely clogged, then heart muscle is damaged or destroyed, leading first to chest pain and then to a full-blown heart attack. For many patients, this meant having a *coronary artery bypass graft* operation done—CABG, or as medical professionals often call it: "cabbage."

Although lifesaving, CABG has been less necessary recently because of a number of medical advances. One advance is angioplasty along with the development of stents, and then stents with drugs attached to them. My point is that these new technologies have reduced the need for CABG surgery. And of course, if we would only improve our lifestyles, there would be less and less coronary artery disease altogether.

FEWER PROCEDURES DONE IN THE HOSPITAL OR

Let's begin by understanding why fewer procedures will need to be done in the hospital operating room. I remember twenty-five years ago when my father needed cataract surgery. He was admitted to the hospital two days before surgery. First, an internist met with him that afternoon and did a complete examination, got a chest X-ray, and did some blood tests. By late the next day, the test results were back and he had been "cleared" for surgery, which was done the following morning, nearly forty-eight hours after his admission. After surgery he was told to lie in bed without moving, with a sandbag up against his face and bandages over his eyes. Finally, the next day, the ophthalmologist removed the bandages, checked his eyes, and discharged him.

Compare that to when my wife's friend had the same surgery last week. She got up in the morning and drove to an ophthalmology outpatient facility with her husband. There she was checked over, had the surgery, and three hours later was back in the car, this time with her husband driving her home, but otherwise she was back to the usual.

Today in a shopping mall nearby, there is a "store" that does another type of eye surgery, this time on the cornea: laser eye surgery, also known as *lasik*. You go in, get tested, the laser surgery is performed, and you come out a short time later without the need for glasses. This is a remarkable surgery and has been of great value to many patients. What I find interesting is that the site for this surgery is not only in the mall, but that a large-screen TV in the window allows passersby to watch the laser surgery in close-up detail. Wow, what marketing!

LESS-INVASIVE SURGERY

You're also aware that many types of surgery are much less invasive today than in the past. The advent of the laparoscope, about twenty years ago, and its many cousins, such as the arthroscope and the thoracoscope, has made huge changes in surgery itself and in the pre- and postoperative preparation. For example, a person who entered the hospital for the removal of his gallbladder (*cholecystectomy*) used to end up with a six-inch incision and about a week postoperative stay. With the laparoscopic technique, only a few one-inch incisions are made in the abdomen and the patient goes home the next morning, sometimes even that afternoon. Laparoscopy can be used for taking out not only the gallbladder, but also for taking out the appendix, doing cancer surgery, removing a kidney, and many other forms of abdominal surgery.

The arthroscope can be used to repair the torn ligament in a "weekend warrior's" knee, rather than using the old open surgery. The thoracoscope can do fairly extensive surgery on the lungs with just some tiny incisions. The results? Less time in the hospital—or even avoiding it altogether in favor of an outpatient center—less pain, less pain medication, faster recuperation, and less opportunity for a hospital-acquired infection or surgical complications.

We are now seeing the introduction of remarkable abilities to do surgical procedures that heretofore required major operative interventions. Consider aortic valve replacement. The aortic valve is the valve between the heart's big pumping chamber and the aorta or big vessel that carries blood to all the major arteries in our body. Sometimes it gets stiff and hard to open and close, with lots of calcium hardening the leaflets of the valve. The repair has been to put the patient on the heart-lung bypass machine, open the chest, stop the heart, open the heart, remove the old valve, and insert a new valve. Lifesaving and greatly improving the quality of everyday life, this has been remarkable surgery.

Within the next five years, you will hear about replacing this valve through the use of a catheter. Remarkable—and it will mean much safer surgery, much shorter hospital stays, and the valve repaired this way may prove to be actually better than the surgically implanted valve—better biomechanics. A real advance.

You can expect hip replacement surgery to become an outpatient procedure soon. Prostate removal for cancer, currently a complex major surgery, will become an outpatient procedure as well. And it will be safer with laparoscopic and robotic technologies.

INTERVENTIONAL RADIOLOGY

One reason fewer procedures will need to be done in the operating room is the rise of interventional radiology.

We tend to think of radiology as taking pictures for diagnosis. But with the ability to see into our bodies and obtain incredibly detailed anatomic pictures immediately, it now becomes possible to do many procedures in the radiology suite that in the past needed to be done with open surgery in the operating room. A good example is diagnostic biopsies. For example, in the past the surgeon made an incision and then removed a segment of the breast, the lung, or other tissue to send to the pathology department.

Today many biopsies are done with image guidance using a needle. If mammography uncovers a suspicious area in the breast, the patient can immediately be taken to the next room where that lesion is biopsied, using a stereo-scopically directed needle. *Stereoscopic* refers to using the image to direct the placement of the biopsy needle. This technique can be incredibly accurate and involves only the needle insertion, rather than an incision, and no stitches. The physician can see when the needle is in place and whether it is exactly where it is wanted, based on the abnormality seen on the image. It's much simpler for the patient than having an open biopsy.

I mentioned aortic aneurysms in an earlier chapter. The aorta is the large artery that comes out of the heart and runs down through the chest and abdomen eventually splitting to run down into both legs. Sometimes, usually in older age, it balloons out in the abdomen. And like any balloon, it can rup-ture or pop. Such an event is catastrophic, so physicians usually recommend that these aneurysms be repaired. It's a big deal.

The surgeon makes a long abdominal incision and then begins to move the stomach and the intestines aside, finally getting to the very back of the abdomen where the aorta is. The surgeon puts clamps across the aorta above and below the diseased area, opens it up, and sews in a graft made of material like Gortex. The clamps are taken off, and the surgery is completed. But more often than not, since this is such extensive surgery, the patient spends four to five or more days in the intensive care unit and then another week or so in the hospital before going home to a prolonged recuperation. Since the individual is frequently older, he or she may also have heart disease, lung disease, or kid-ney disease, any of which can make the surgery much riskier and the postop-erative period more prone to complications.

But contrast that to what can be done for many patients today in the inter-ventional radiology suite. The patient is put into a drowsy state with some medication and then a catheter is inserted into the big artery in the groin. The catheter is threaded up to the area in the aorta where the aneurysm is, all of which can be seen with the imaging techniques. Using the catheter, a graft (tubing) can be inserted on the inside of the aorta, hooked down to the walls of the aorta, and the catheter removed. Total time may be an hour and a half, and after staying in the hospital overnight for observation, the patient can go home.

I recently met a lovely seventy-eight-year-old man with a huge aortic aneurysm. Clearly, this was a time bomb ticking away. But he also had signif-icant heart disease and lung disease, so no surgeon would risk doing open surgery. He was a perfect candidate for the new technology, which went smoothly. I saw him when he was coming back for his six-month checkup with his surgeon. He brought with him a photograph of himself and his wife at his birthday party the week before. He still has his heart and lung problems, but he won't die from a burst aneurysm.

Here's another example. There are three major types of strokes, the most common being the development of a blood clot that blocks the flow of blood in one of the major arteries either to or in the brain. The second possibility is that a clot moves up to the brain from somewhere else in the body, such as from the heart. And the third cause of stroke is when an artery in the brain develops an aneurysm, a ballooning out, and then begins to bleed. These can be truly devastating strokes.

A forty-four-year-old woman, whom I will call Rhonda Perkins, seemingly in perfectly good health, suddenly developed what she called the worst headache of her life. Fairly quickly she was having weakness in her right arm and leg and some difficulty speaking. Her husband called her internist who easily enough diagnosed a developing stroke over the telephone. He also knew that the severe headache most certainly meant that she had an aneurysm that was starting to bleed. So he immediately arranged for her to be transported to a major medical center, which fortunately was only a half hour from their home. She was met at the medical center by members of the "brain attack" team.

As a side note, the term *stroke* is often called *brain attack* in an attempt by physicians to get people to realize that it needs immediate attention, just like a heart attack. This is no time to wait around to see if the symptoms get better. Immediate diagnosis and treatment may prevent lasting brain damage.

The examination and imaging quickly confirmed the diagnosis. The usual approach in such a situation would be for a neurosurgeon to take the patient to the operating room, open the skull, and with delicate surgery get to the spot where the aneurysm is located. Then the neurosurgeon would place silver clips across the aneurysm so that it could no longer bleed. The surgery saves lives, especially if it can be done quickly enough after the aneurysm begins to cause symptoms. But it's also an extremely delicate major surgery.

Usually the patient is in the neurosurgical intensive care unit for a number of days and then in the hospital for observation before going home or to rehabilitation. But this lady was more fortunate. She was taken to the neuroradiology suite where the neurosurgeon and radiologist, working together, took a different approach. Like the patient described previously, she was put into a drowsy state with medication, and then a catheter was inserted into that same major artery in her groin. This time it was threaded up through the aorta in the abdomen, through the aorta in the chest, then into the carotid artery that goes up through the neck to the brain, and finally to the middle cerebral artery, deep within the brain.

The aneurysm could be seen on the imaging device. It looked like a small balloon, perhaps the size of the end of your little finger, sticking out from the artery. The catheter was turned and inserted right into the aneurysm. Then multiple tiny platinum coils were inserted into the aneurysm through the catheter. These coils cause blood to clot around them. After the aneurysm was filled with the platinum coils and the blood had clotted, the aneurysm was no more. The whole procedure took about an hour and forty-five minutes. The only incision was about a quarter-inch long in her groin.

Mrs. Perkins never saw the inside of an operating room. But her aneurysm was cured. After a few days in the hospital she was sent to a rehabilitation center where—with the diligent help of physical and speech therapists, along with her own hard work—she regained full use of her arm and leg and, unless you listen carefully, her speech sounds perfect today.

So what else can be done in the interventional radiology suite? We have already discussed coronary artery angioplasty and stent placements. Here are a few other examples. Sometimes a patient has colon cancer that has spread to the liver in such a way that there is just one large mass in the liver. If it's at one end or the other the surgeon can remove that entire segment of the liver and throw away that big tumor. Sounds simple, but it is really a major, complex, delicate surgery. But if you have a superb surgeon, it works, and in the next six weeks the liver will grow back to its former size.

If the tumor has developed in the middle of the liver, such surgery is not possible. But in the interventional radiology suite, a device can be inserted directly through the abdominal or chest wall into the middle of the cancer, all under the guidance of the imaging machines. Then, using radio frequency waves, the tumor can be heated to the point where all the cancer cells are killed. Since the liver has such a rapid blood flow, the normal tissue away from the area that's being heated is cooled by the flowing blood so that only the tumor itself and a surrounding area of normal tissue will be destroyed.

For example, a gentleman was referred to a gastroenterologist because of liver failure. It turned out that his liver failure resulted from the hepatitis C virus. He had become infected some twenty years before, when he had had open-heart surgery to correct a congenital defect. He had been given blood transfusions before the development of a test to detect and eliminate donors who carried the virus. It's a virus that hangs around in the liver, often for life, and slowly but surely damages the liver.

Now, twenty years later, he had severe damage called *cirrhosis*. Because he was otherwise healthy, he was a clear candidate for a liver transplant. Without the transplant he would certainly die. But while waiting for a liver to become available (usually a multiyear wait, and more people die while on the waiting list than actually ever get a liver transplant), he developed a new problem. In the middle of his liver was a baseball-sized mass. A needle biopsy, inserted through the abdomen and into the mass, revealed *hepatoma*, a type of cancer.

Hepatomas are a relatively uncommon form of cancer, but they are often caused by hepatitis C, occurring in people who also have hepatitis-induced liver failure. The tumor was growing rapidly, and it would potentially kill him before his liver failed and before a transplant could be found. It was not amenable to surgery because of its location, so the radio frequency ablation technique was tried. Everything seemed fine, but the images taken some weeks later to see if the tumor had disappeared showed something still there. But it stopped growing, and it started to shrink.

Then miraculously a liver became available and he received the transplant. After the old liver was taken out, pathologists carefully sectioned it to see what was left of the hepatoma. All that was left was some scar tissue and some dead and necrotic cells. The RF ablation technique had worked perfectly and destroyed the entire tumor. Meanwhile the gentleman is doing fine following his liver transplant.

Here's another example of the use of interventional radiology. A small proportion of people who have elevated blood pressure are found to have *renal artery stenosis*. This means that the artery coming from the aorta to the kidney has a constriction along it, which can cause a rise in blood pressure that usually won't respond well to drug therapy. This stenosis can be corrected by surgery. The surgeon goes through the same steps that I described for the aortic aneurysm example, and reaching the artery to the kidney, replaces the constricted segment with a graft. Sounds simple, but again, it's major surgery.

Now, just like putting a stent into a coronary artery, a physician can insert a catheter into the groin, pass it up the aorta, turn it into the renal artery (the artery to the kidney), and having found the narrowed area, open it with the balloon, followed by a stent to keep it open. The procedure is reasonably easy to do by an experienced operator and is certainly much easier on the patient than open surgery. As usual, I use the words *easy* or *minor* with some trepidation. It is still a highly technical procedure that requires great skill and much experience. It should be performed only by an expert in an institution where the procedure is done frequently.

These are just some of the ways in which procedures can be done today without the need for an operating room or major incisions. Recovery time is obviously much faster and pain is reduced, as are complications. In the coming years we will see many more advances of this type that will allow treatment without the need for the open surgery of the past. Interventional radiology is another of those disruptive technologies—and as new ideas and approaches are employed, these technologies will continue to disrupt the way we practice medicine today and transform it into a better, simpler, and safer medicine of the future.

EXTENDED FUNCTIONALITY OF THE OPERATING ROOM

Now let's turn to what I call the *extended functionality* of the operating room of the future. Use your imagination again. A large hospital might have, say, twenty operating rooms.

Each room gets used, for example, an average of three times a day. Some, of course, might have seven or eight relatively short procedures done, and others might have one patient in the room for an entire day. But let's just go with the averages. Twenty rooms times three procedures means sixty cases per day. Each case requires the correct sterile instrument tray and the correct equipment, such as laparoscopes. The room has to be staffed with nurses and scrub technicians who are familiar with the case. The anesthesia staff needs to be scheduled. And of course the various surgeons need to know when their cases are scheduled to begin. Housekeeping needs to be properly scheduled so that each room can be cleaned and readied quickly between cases, so as to not lose any time.

And let's not forget the patients. There are sixty of them, and they each have to be brought to the correct operating room at the correct time. If you think about it, this is a logistical nightmare! Indeed, it is truly amazing that these large suites of operating rooms function every day as well as they do.

They function because of a nurse manager, surgical medical director, and anesthesia medical director working hard together. The directors are constantly being called to find some equipment for this room, get an anesthesiologist for that room, and figure out why all the instruments in a third room aren't there. Usually it means running up and down the hall all day. But some simple advances help this troika today.

Giving them cell phones that work inside the hospital means they can communicate with each other without running up and down the hall, and they can call central sterile supply or the equipment room from wherever they are. Cameras can be placed in each operating room and each room can be observed through a central console, similar to the way security guards watch monitors from cameras placed at various locations. They can see if the equipment is in the room, if the room has been cleaned and readied for the next patient, and if the instrument tray is there, opened and ready to go. And for that matter, they can tell if the surgeon, anesthesiologist, nurse, and patient are all there. Add to this wireless technology, and our three managers can carry a "Palm Pilot" so they can see into any of the multiple operating rooms from any location.

At the central nursing desk in every suite of operating rooms is the "white board" where the staff lists each room, the patient who is in each room, the type of surgery that's scheduled, the names of the surgeons, the anesthesiologist, and the scrub nurse or technician. When a case has been completed, that information can be erased and the name of the next patient, type of surgery, and so forth, can be entered. It's a simple yet effective device for managing the operating room and seeing at a glance what's going on in each OR. Video cameras can be of assistance here as well.

Instead of looking at the white board and then moving over to where the centralized video monitors are located, it's now possible to have the video image projected right onto the white board on a section next to each room number. Now the three managers can read not only what's going on in each room, but they can actually see concurrently what the state of activity is. Is the patient on the table? Has surgery begun? Has surgery ended? Has the room been cleaned? All can be seen at a glance for every operating room.

After these video white board images had been in place for a few months, the chief of surgery of a major trauma center told me that they made his life much easier. In the past, he would routinely go into each operating room for a few moments to see the status of each surgery. Now he can check the white board in just a few seconds and can easily do it multiple times a day. He told me this helps him dramatically as he tries to balance which trauma patient in urgent need of surgery can get to the next available operating room.

Just as these devices help in the management of the operating room suites, they also can assist the surgeon, anesthesiologist, and nurse in their care of the patients. With better information technology, Internet access, and wireless capabilities, all of the patient's critical information can be instantly available. Most patients today, unfortunately, have their information spread over multiple sites. First, the surgeon saw them in his office, and those notes were almost undoubtedly handwritten and probably not entered into a computerized system.

Then the patient was evaluated before surgery by the anesthesiologist. And that information is somewhere. Results of blood and urine tests and X-rays that were taken before surgery are somewhere else. Now it's the day of surgery, and that information usually is not all there in the paper record available in the operating room. As electronic medical record keeping develops, all this information will be available, regardless of where it was obtained. The technology is available today to have a computer screen and keyboard on a mobile cart in the operating room, working by wireless technology to collect data from any part of the electronic medical record, directly or via the Internet for off-site information.

One day soon, health care providers will access all of the images that had been obtained in the past, all the laboratory data, and all the physicians' and nurses' notes that were in the record already. Unfortunately, most of this information is not available electronically today. In fact, most of the information technology in the operating room today could probably be described as a "disabler," as it's not designed for the health care professional, but rather for OR managers who need information for staffing and scheduling.

As a result, professionals spend all too much of their time in nonprofessional activities, such as transporting patients and materials. Further, the operating room itself generates a lot of information from the various monitors, such as pulse rate, blood pressure, and oxygenation of the blood. For the surgeon and anesthesiologist, this information is scattered about the OR. Just as the "white board" at the entrance to the OR suite helps staff in their planning and activities, an electronic white board within the OR itself is proving useful.

Recognizing that a data glut can result in chaos, the data—via some artificial intelligence concepts—is being reduced, selected, simplified, and presented in a useful manner on a video screen in the OR. This offers surgeons, anesthesiologists, and nurses an improved *situational awareness.* Situational awareness sounds like a big phrase, but for these three professionals in the OR, it is all-important. They need to know—*now*—the status of their patient so they can make appropriate course corrections as they proceed, especially in long, complex cases.

Even the architecture of the operating room is changing. As the OR becomes increasingly complex, as the pace becomes faster, as the amount of equipment grows exponentially, and the instruments become more varied, more and better organized space is needed. The ORs of just a few years ago were four hundred square feet; now they're being built at six to seven hundred square feet. Instead of having lots of equipment on the floor or on carts, all this equipment can be suspended from booms that hang from the ceiling. This means less stuff on the OR floor, which means less likelihood of staff members tripping, and it's much easier to clean the OR between cases.

During laparoscopic surgery, the surgeon depends upon a video screen to see what he or she is doing. Instead of having a bulky TV on a cart in the room, multiple flat-panel screens hang from the ceiling and the surgeon can easily reposition them to best advantage. The anesthesiologist and nurse can have their own screen and now see the same things that the surgeon sees throughout the operation, increasing their ability to help. The operating room has more and better lights and much better air circulation, which is not only more comfortable, but also reduces the chance for infection. Instead of making changes to equipment by foot pedals, hand cranks, or switches, now voice activation can turn the lights up, the temperature down, adjust the head or foot of the operating table, and even select suitable music to play in the OR that seems best for the case at hand.

One thing that slows down work in the operating room is that many activities are done serially—a long-standing tradition—rather than at the same time. Massachusetts General Hospital in Boston has taken an area and completely reconfigured both the architecture and the way things work. Instead of an OR being one room, there are now three interconnected rooms—a room to start the anesthesia, the OR itself, and a room to start the recovery process. Instead of putting the patient to sleep in the operating room, it's done in the adjacent anesthesia induction room. This can be done while the operating room is being cleaned and restocked.

Then the patient is brought in for the start of surgery and when surgery is over is moved to the other small room where postanesthesia recovery begins. This again gets the patient out of the OR so that cleaning and restocking can start. The surgical team using this room for reasonably straightforward laparoscopic abdominal surgery finds that they can do an average of 6.4 cases per day, compared to the previous 5.3. And they can do those additional cases in an average of 8.6 hours, instead of 9.5 hours. For example, a gallbladder removal that used to take 104 minutes now takes 74 minutes, done by the same surgeon, anesthesiologist, and nurse, using the same equipment.

Technology is another element of the extended functionality of the operating room of the future. A big change is *intraoperative imaging*. For years, it has been possible to take an X-ray immediately after the surgeon does a procedure or part of a procedure. For example, an orthopedist might want to see how bones are lined up after doing a repair and takes an X-ray before completing the surgery. Obviously, it's best to do this while the patient is still asleep and in the operating room.

Sophisticated X-ray equipment built into the surgical suite is another big advance, such as in neurosurgery where *angiograms* (injecting a dye into a vessel and then taking multiple pictures, similar to a movie, as the dye runs through the vessels in the brain) can check the state of the surgery. Here again, this can help the surgeon not only in planning, but also in checking the surgery as it goes along.

Then along came *neuronavigation*. A CAT scan or an MRI is taken before surgery. The images, all digital, are loaded into a computerized device in the operating room. On the monitor screen the surgeon can see either slices of various levels of the brain from the CAT scan or MRI or can convert them into a three-dimensional virtual picture of the brain. Let's say that the surgeon is removing a brain tumor. The surgeon is working through a relatively small opening often deep inside brain tissue. All of the tumor must be removed, but not any more normal brain than necessary, since it might affect how a person walks, talks, or functions after surgery.

Even the best neurosurgeons will tell you that when working within these confines, it can be very difficult to tell where the edge of the tumor is and where the normal brain begins. With the neuronavigation device, the surgeon can see the tumor and the normal brain on a computer screen. Now for the "Buck Rogers" part. This neuronavigation device, through infrared and other technologies, can detect within a millimeter or two where the surgeon's scalpel or probe or other device is in the brain. It then shows this on the computer screen relative to the MRI or CAT scan that was done before surgery.

This makes the surgery much more accurate and allows the surgeon to have a much greater level of confidence that the tumor has been fully removed. As one superb neurosurgeon said to me, "This will make a good surgeon better, but it won't make a bad surgeon good."

All of these techniques make the OR safer for the patient, more functional for the staff, and allow a highly expensive resource to be used most efficiently.

A ROOM WITH A NEW VIEW

With these changes in mind, let's turn to the room with a new view. Let's begin to think five, ten, and fifteen years from now. To do so, we first have to understand laparoscopic surgery and how imaging is transforming surgical practice.

Room with a New View

- Less Invasive Surgery
- Video Devices on Wall and in Light Source
- Simulators
- Robotics
- ID Devices for Instruments, Equipment, Staff and Patient
- Surgeon Practices on Virtual Specific Patient

Laparoscopic Surgery and Image Guidance

This revolutionary surgery, twenty years old now, continues to change medicine today. Let me oversimplify it with an example of removing a gallbladder.

In the past, a six- to eight-inch incision would have been made in the abdomen, so that the surgeon and the assistant could reach in and—using a scalpel, forceps, and other equipment—isolate the relevant structures, clamp off the blood supply to the gallbladder, check for stones in the common bile duct, and remove the gallbladder. It was a common and relatively straightforward operation in most patients, but it did mean about a week in the hospital and some weeks for recovery afterward.

With laparoscopic surgery a small incision, about half an inch, is made in the abdomen and a device about as big around as a lead pencil with a tiny camera on the end is inserted. Carbon dioxide is pumped into the abdomen to puff up a space so that the surgeon can see and work, all based on what pictures the camera sends back to the screen in the operating room. Then one or two other small incisions are made and surgeons insert long-handled instruments, again with diameters about the size of a large pencil. On the far inside end will be tools, such as clamps or cutting devices like scissors, and on the outside end will be handles that allow the surgeon to manipulate those tools.

Try to imagine that you're the surgeon for a moment. In the older "open" approach, the surgeon could see everything, including the gallbladder and the blood vessels. The surgeon could also touch those tissues and organs and had a good sense through touch and sight of what was happening and what was being done. In laparoscopic surgery, everything happens through visualization on a monitor. The surgeon does not have direct sight and does not have any sense of touch. The instrument head with its tools is a few feet away from his or her hands that are holding on to the handles of this long device. If you were to observe laparoscopic surgery, you might be struck by the fact that no one is looking at the patient! Instead everyone is looking at the TV screen. It's sort of an eerie sight when you first see it. Now the surgeon is dependent on images and is "disconnected" from any direct visual contact with the tissue.

Since the surgeon is now visualizing tissue based on a camera and a monitor, it's possible to digitize this information and manipulate it, as we will discuss later. Bottom line, imaging has become increasingly important in the operating room, and not just the image that the surgeon can see through the laparoscope, but images that can be taken before or during surgery by the increasingly sophisticated CAT scans, MRI, and other technologies.

Every surgeon will tell you that he or she does not want to have any surprises during an operation. No two people have exactly the same anatomy, but if you look at anatomy books, what is shown is "the average," or occasionally the most common differences among people. But the surgeon would like to know in advance *exactly* what's going to be found and where.

Let's consider what happened when Mr. McClellan needed a kidney transplant. In his early fifties, he began to develop chronic kidney failure. It wasn't entirely clear to his physicians why this began, although he did have high blood pressure that was reasonably controlled by medications. His kidney failure had reached the point where he needed dialysis with all the trials and tribulations and potential complications that come with its lifesaving potential. He was placed on the waiting list for a kidney transplant, but knew that most people who got a transplant have been on the waiting list for upward of two to three years.[1]

Mr. McClellan's son, in his early thirties, volunteered to donate one of his kidneys. Mr. McClellan was initially opposed. He was told that having only one kidney would be more than adequate for his son. But he also thought that he would feel incredibly guilty and would always worry that perhaps his son would develop some type of kidney problem himself in the years to come. Having only one kidney in such a situation would put him at a significant medical disadvantage. But his son insisted and eventually he agreed.

Only a few years ago, donating a kidney was not only a lifesaving gift, but also major surgery for the donor. A long incision would be made in the flank, the kidney would be removed, the incision would be sewn up, and the donor would probably stay in the hospital four to five days with substantial pain, followed by about a six-week recuperation period at home. It would mean substantial time off from work or from activities at home. The combination of the pain and the long recuperation time was certainly a dissuader from volunteering to donate.

Then along came the laparoscopic approach to kidney removal. An incision is made in the *umbilicus* (belly button) area, where the scar will probably never be seen, along with one or two other small incisions. All the work is done through these, including clamping off the artery to the kidney and letting the blood drain out, then clamping off the vein and removing the kidney into a small plastic bag similar to the plastic baggie you use at home for sandwiches, which is then pulled out through the small incision in the umbilicus. It's quite amazing that the kidney, when the blood is drained out, shrinks down enough that it can come out through that small incision. The recovery time is a few days in the hospital, the discomfort is much less, and after only a few days at home the donor is back to work, or perhaps decides to take a well-deserved vacation. This approach to removing the kidney certainly makes it easier for someone to volunteer as a donor.

But wait—there is more to be considered. The surgeon who is going to transplant the donated kidney into Mr. McClellan wants to have the donated kidney removed with as much artery and as much vein as possible, so there is room to work and sew things in. In general this would mean taking the kidney from the right side, but surgically that's more difficult because of the presence of the liver. The surgeon removing a kidney would rather work from the left side with no liver in the way, but the artery and vein on that side will probably be shorter. Sometimes, there's not just one artery, but two or even three arteries to the kidney. It sure would be nice to know this well in advance of the surgery so that appropriate decisions could be made before starting.

One way to find out is to insert a catheter into the large artery in the groin and push it up into the aorta, past the area where the arteries to the kidneys come off, and inject the dye and take X-rays. This will show how the blood vessels go into the kidneys and come back out. But inserting a catheter into a perfectly healthy donor is different than inserting a catheter into someone who has a disease. Any procedure has a risk and you'd like to reduce the risks to the donor as much as possible. New CT scanners are up to the job. With their ability to show three-dimensional models of the vessels, the surgeon can see exactly what vessels come off the aorta and go to each kidney, how many there are, and how long they are. Now a truly rational decision about surgery can be made in advance.

Mr. McClellan's son had the CAT scan taken, the blood vessels to his kidneys were checked out, and at the same time it was possible to study both kidneys to see that they had no cysts or other damage. The surgery proceeded successfully, and as a result, Mr. McClellan was given the gift of life by his son. He returned to his job within a few days, and Mr. McClellan is back at his job as well.

Every day it seems that laparoscopic technology is improving.

Recent improvements include the ability to visualize better, thanks to new flat-screen monitors that have greater resolution and better cameras that can see at a wider angle, yet with sharper focus and much improved color. Soon surgeons will be able to see three-dimensional images in the operative field. Work is going on in the field of *haptics*—the ability to feel even while working through an instrument that's about two feet long.

During the coming years, new ways of imaging will evolve, and those images will be available in real time, giving the surgeon the ability to "see" inside the body in ways almost undreamed of today. As one technology sees better in one dimension, another technology may see better in another dimension. An example of this today is the CT scan and the PET scanner. In an earlier chapter we talked about how the CT scanner looks at anatomy, whereas the PET scanner looks at function or metabolism.

In recent years, it's been possible to make combined scanners that take both a CT image and a PET image and then fuse the two images together. This type of image fusion, using new technologies plus the old technologies, will allow for multimodality imaging in the future. In the near future, the surgeon will be able to see the tumor and its edges clearly with some combination of CT or MRI plus PET. The tumor's lymphatic drainage will be detected perhaps by CT scanning, and its blood supply again by a CT or angiography.

All of this will be integrated to give a total picture only dreamed about until recently.

So far, we've talked about how laparoscopic surgery works and how it separates the surgeon from the site of surgery. We have discussed how, through new imaging and visualization technologies and through the developing field of haptics, it's increasingly possible to put the surgeon back at the site of surgery and give the surgeon much more information than was possible in the former open surgical field. Now let's consider how we can use some of this acquired imaging data for simulation.

Surgical Simulation

I was on a plane a few years ago flying from Denver to Baltimore. Toward the end of the flight, I put my work away in my briefcase and stowed it under the seat, at which point the gentleman sitting next to me struck up a conversation. It turned out he was a senior pilot for United Airlines and the route he flew was Newark, New Jersey, to Tokyo, Japan. He explained that he lived on the Eastern Shore of Maryland and would fly up to Newark where he would captain a Boeing 747 nonstop to Tokyo. Once he arrived in Tokyo, he was required to spend a number of days resting and getting over jetlag before beginning the return flight. When he returned, he had a long hiatus before he flew the next flight.

Unlike in his younger days flying a 737 with multiple take-offs and landings each day, he now did only a few take-offs and landings each month. This explained why he was also flying from Denver to Baltimore. He had been in Denver at the United Airlines Simulation Center where for two days he had practiced more than a dozen take-offs and landings with multiple simulated emergencies, weather issues, and so on. He explained that it had been a great experience, almost exactly as though he were in the cockpit of his Tokyo-bound 747, and that it gave him the opportunity to maintain his skills.

Using simulators for operating room practice is not commonplace; however, I am sure that it will become routine in the coming years. Today, simulators for the operating room are nowhere nearly as advanced as they are for the airline industry, even though a variety of simulators is available. The military has developed simulators to train medics to insert chest tubes; simulators allow for practice inserting a tube into the airway while others simulate starting IV lines.

I had the opportunity to try out a limited laparoscopic simulator. The device looked like a box with a rubberlike cover that was meant to represent the abdominal wall. The laparoscopic instruments passed through a number of half-inch slits in the wall. One instrument held the miniaturized camera that projected onto a TV screen in front of me, and the other instrument held a set of pinchers. Inside the abdomen were five small round dishes. In one of the dishes were four marbles. My task was to move the laparoscopic pinchers into the dish with the marbles, grab a marble, lift it out of the dish, and then place it in one of the other dishes. This was repeated until there was a marble in each of the four dishes.

Having never handled any type of laparoscopic instrument before, I can tell you that this was something of a challenge. Within a few minutes though, I was able to grasp the marbles and move them to the various dishes. I was rather proud of myself, but the simulator gave me a poor score. "Why?" I questioned the instructor who was standing beside me.

"Well," she said, smiling, "you got them from the one dish to the other dishes, but it took you five minutes, whereas it would take an experienced surgeon less than thirty seconds. Second, you got them there, but the simulator monitored your hand motions. Look at this graph on the monitor, you were certainly not smooth. The idea is to move them in a very smooth movement; yours were not."

Now, I'm not a surgeon, but I do have reasonable dexterity, and what I took away from this rather limited example is that every medical student should have the same experience I had and every surgical resident should have to demonstrate a high level of competence on this and other simulation devices before ever being allowed to assist in laparoscopic surgery in the operating room. That's exactly what is happening in some medical centers around the country. Yes, the current simulators are still relatively crude, but they are improving every year. Trainees who have the opportunity to work with them almost invariably say that it was a major help in learning to do laparoscopic surgery.

One of the advantages of a simulator is that you get immediate feedback, as I did in my limited experiment.

These will become routine and ultimately use images acquired from the specific patient, enabling the surgeon to practice the exact surgery needed for that person. No one questions that simulators will be fundamental to surgical training. But simulators have a long way to go before they will have the ability to model tissue properties. For example, in open surgery the surgeon can touch and feel a tissue. Surgeons will tell you that when tying a knot in a suture, part of the technique is getting a sense of the tension on the suture and the tissue. Too much tension and the tissue can be torn; too little tension and the suture knot will not be tight.

Simulators also need realistic portrayals of bleeding, so that the trainee can deal with this in the simulated environment. Virtual patient training technology eventually can be based upon the patient's own digitized images, or at least a digitized representative patient. In time, interactive holography and three-dimensional computers will simulate complex movements and positions. These aren't available yet, but they're coming.

Like any new technology, sometimes there's a reluctance to get involved. Some surgeons say that the only way to train is on a live patient and resist using the simulator. But with time they will learn to appreciate that the most complex and difficult aspects of the surgery can be practiced on the simulator without doing all the other elements of the procedure. This is like the pilot who practiced take-off and landings with the simulator in Denver, but not too many of the other elements of a fourteen-hour flight.

Sometimes it's regulatory bodies that force the adoption of new techniques and technologies. I mentioned earlier that a new stent recently became available for use in the carotid artery. The carotid artery is that large artery that runs up from the chest through the neck to the brain and it can get clogged with plaque just like a coronary artery. And as in doing angioplasty and stenting of a coronary artery, one can insert a stent into the carotid artery. But when the Food and Drug Administration approved a new stent in 2005, the FDA added a requirement that only a physician who had demonstrated competency on the affiliated simulator could insert the stent.

I talked to a vascular surgeon friend of mine who has been inserting stents for almost ten years. He told me that the new stent is much better, but he particularly enjoyed using the simulator. He found that the feel was similar to what it felt like when inserting the stent in an actual patient. He was able to practice multiple times, and therefore felt that he had a good grasp of how this particular stent worked and how it worked in a typical carotid artery. He felt that the FDA had made a wise decision and hoped this would lead to similar requirements for other uses of simulators.

Simulators aren't just for practicing surgical techniques. For example, efforts are being made to develop a virtual work flow simulator for the operating room. It takes a lot of practice and effort to make all the activities within the operating room—before, during, and after surgery—work smoothly. By simulating these efforts in a virtual reality setting, it is possible for each member of the team to practice his or her part. Get the room cleaned. Then get it stocked with equipment and instruments for the next case. Then be sure that the patient (and the medical staff) is available, has been premedicated, and brought to the operating room. After surgery, the patient must be transferred to a recovery room and follow-up steps need to be done. Working all this through on a simulator not only allows practice, but also detects difficulties and allows the staff to create a more effective and efficient set of processes.

Are there other approaches to improving surgical skills? You might be a little bit distressed if you learned that your surgeon was an avid video game player. You might think that he or she should spend more time worrying about surgery instead of playing games. Some interesting preliminary information indicates that surgeons who "warm up" with a video game before surgery actually perform better surgery. Perhaps we can liken it to a golfer going to the driving range and the putting green before stepping onto the golf course for the real game.

Simulation

- Stent Placement
- Chest Tube Insertion
- IV Line Insertion
- Laparoscopic Instrument Practice and Evaluation of Operator/ Trainee
- Surgical/ Anesthesia Crises Practice
- Team Building/ Team Experiences
- Work Flow Simulation
- Presurgery Design of Optimal Operation
- Role of Video Games in Practice

At a conference recently, I learned that the surgical residents who warmed up with some video game time were found, in a simulated environment, to have 32 percent fewer errors, to be 24 percent faster, and to have an overall 26 percent better score on a standardized procedure. Considering this, should you ask your surgeon just before being put to sleep if she did well on her video game before breakfast this morning?

Bottom line: Simulation will have an exceptionally important role in medicine in the future. Not just in surgery but in all procedure training. And not just for physicians, but also for nurses, technicians, and others. Indeed, training in medicine will fundamentally change. Simulators will be available for all types of procedure learning and practice. And the requirements for certification will change. Instead of needing to have completed X number of procedures before being approved, a physician will need to demonstrate competency on the simulator for that procedure. For some, it may take many practice runs to become competent; for others, fewer runs may be required. But the measure will be competence—as it should be.

Teaching hospitals will need to change what they consider to be critical elements of the learning and training processes. Hospital executives will need to accept that the purchase of simulators and staffing of simulation laboratories will be not only routine, but also mandatory. And faculty physicians will need to become proficient in using simulators for training the next generation of health care providers. This will be a momentous culture change in how we train physicians and others, but it will come—and quickly. The result will be better surgery, more effective surgery, and much safer surgery. And, although I have dealt with simulation in the OR chapter, this is a transformational megatrend that will affect all branches of medicine—the cardiologist doing catheterizations, the gastroenterologist doing a colonoscopy, the interventionalist putting in an aortic aneurysm graft, or the medical student learning to draw blood from a vein. All of medical education and training will change over the coming years—a major change for the better.

Robotic Surgery

I used the term *robotic surgery* in the story at the beginning of this chapter. But the concept of robots in surgery is actually quite different than the autonomous or semiautonomous R2D2 of science fiction and the movies, and it differs from the industrial robots of, for example, an auto assembly plant. A better term might be *remote computer-assisted telemanipulators*. This is quite a mouthful, but what it basically means is to merge industrial robotic technology with three-dimensional visualization systems and computer technology.

Two of the arms of the robotic device can hold and move instruments, such as laparoscopic instruments, and a third arm can transmit two independent images from a stereo telescopic camera mounted at its tip. Remember the discussion of the laparoscopic instrument? It's a long rod with, for example, a pincher device at one end, which will be inside the abdomen, and a set of handles to operate the pincher at the far external end of the laparoscope. The amount of freedom of movement in the laparoscopic instrument is rather limited.

Compare that to the surgeon doing open surgery whose arm, wrist, and hand is within the abdominal cavity. We speak of the wrist as having six degrees of freedom of movement—look at your wrist and watch how you can move it up, down, left, right, and in a rotational motion either direction. The laparoscopic device is much more limited. The joints and arms of the robotic surgical devices also have six degrees of freedom of movement. If these devices are inside the patient and attached to the robot rather than being held in the surgeon's hands, how does the surgeon control the system?

The answer is that the surgeon's head sits inside a console in which he or she can see a three-dimensional image of the operative field, created by integration of the right and left camera images, within the console. So the surgeon has a clear three-dimensional view of the robotic surgery and can manipulate tissue with the instruments as if the surgeon's hands were holding the laparoscopic instruments inside the patient. This is done by having the surgeon hold a series of handles at the console to manipulate the robotic arms. The surgeon is fully in control of the equipment.

One definite downside to the equipment today is that the surgeon does not get any sense of what the robotic arm is "feeling," that is, no tactile feedback or haptics. Other disadvantages are cost—these systems currently cost more than $1 million each—and their large size makes them hard to move.

But it is a remarkable advance, and it's being used today in cardiac and prostate surgery with good results. Watch for advertisements in which a local hospital is trying to show they're more advanced than the competition by touting that they have these robotic systems in their center. My advice would be to remember what the neurosurgeon told me about neuronavigation: "This will make a good surgeon better, but it won't make a bad surgeon good." It's

Robotic Surgery

- ■ "Remote Computer Assisted Telemanipulators"
- ■ Surgeon Works from Console
- ■ Joints with "6 Degrees of Freedom"
- ■ Improve Efficacy
- ■ Improve Safety

the same for robotic surgery; it can assist a good, experienced surgeon, but in the hands of a novice, it will make for potential disasters. What's most important to you as a potential patient or relative is to be sure that the surgeon is well trained with lots of experience and a great track record. Then if he or she plans to use the robot on you, ask how much experience the surgeon has had with it, and with what kind of results, including complications.

The current robotic equipment is certainly costly, but like any other new technology, I assume the price will drop and that ultimately robotic devices will help to lower rather than raise surgical costs. It should enable new, less-invasive approaches to surgery. Surgical acceptance will be uneasy at first, if only because these devices require the development of a new set of skills. This includes the use of multimodality imaging, which is much different from direct visualization or the type of visualization a surgeon gets in classic laparoscopic surgery today. Second, this type of surgery really is guided by preoperative procedure planning, which is not the norm in surgical settings today. Third, the surgery itself is guided by intraoperative guidance software; in other words, the surgeon is being assisted in making the right maneuvers.

As the combination of robotics and simulation takes hold, expect teams of surgeons and others to work together from disparate locations, such as different hospitals with surgeons of different skills and expertise, to model in advance the design of an operation for a difficult situation. They will do it in virtual reality, and then the patient's surgeon will use this developed plan to perform the surgery with the aid of the robot.

I mentioned that these robotic devices are being used today at some centers for cardiac surgery. Now I'd like to invite you to use your imagination again. A patient is put on the heart-lung bypass machine, so that during cardiac surgery the heart can be stopped to allow the surgeon to work without the heart beating. Obviously it's difficult to suture a vein bypass to a coronary artery while the heart is beating. But what if the robot was so sophisticated that it could use the electrocardiogram to tell it when the heart will beat? Then the robot's arms could be adjusted electronically to the beating heart, so that the arm of the robot and the instrument that the robot is holding are all moving the same as the heart is moving.

In essence this would give the appearance that the heart was standing still as the surgeon watches the effort on the three-dimensional console screen. Now the surgeon can do precise suturing on a beating heart rather than a heart that has been stopped. This, of course, means that the heart-lung machine, with all of its potential for complications, wouldn't be necessary.

Some types of surgery, especially laparoscopic surgery, are ergonomically taxing on the surgeon and assistants, meaning that it is difficult, for example, to hold the laparoscope in one position for long periods of time. In time, minimally invasive surgery will gravitate more toward robotics, if only to improve ergonomics. The robot's arm or hand, obviously, doesn't get tired. Robots can also be programmed to avoid certain structures during a procedure—so the possibility of an error is greatly reduced. This concept is being called setting "no fly zones" such as assuring that the robotic arms cannot move and cut a nerve, for example, during prostate surgery.

Another use of robotics is as a surgical scrub technician. A device developed at Columbia-Presbyterian Hospital in New York called *Penelope* can listen for voice commands, pick up the desired instrument, hand it to the surgeon, and then retrieve it after the surgeon is done. Penelope keeps track of everything from instruments to whether all the sponges have been retrieved from the abdomen. This will improve not only inventory control, but safety as well since a sponge, for example, cannot be left behind by mistake.

Not too long ago, a gallbladder removal was done in France using a surgical robot. But the surgeon, Dr. Jacques Marescaux, was not at the console in the operating room, but at a console in New York! So this was *transatlantic telerobotic laparoscopic cholecystectomy*. Let's just call it *telesurgery* for short. What could this mean for the future?

Imagine someone needing urgent surgery in a remote location where a trained surgeon is not available. Or imagine a soldier wounded on the battlefield, who needs a particular type of surgery, but the expert is oceans away. In both cases telesurgery could make the needed surgery available.

Dr. Mehran Anvari, a surgeon in Canada, has performed several telesurgeries, operating from his hospital suite in Hamilton, Ontario, on patients in a hospital in North Bay, a distance of about five hundred miles. A reliable telephone line and solid communications with physicians in North Bay have ensured the success of all of these surgeries and allowed the expertise of Dr. Anvari to be applied to patient care from a great distance.

Recently, in a research project sponsored by NASA, the Canadian Space Agency, and TATRC, Dr. Anvari, performed surgical skill tasks in Canada on a simulated patient located in the NOAA underwater laboratory off the coast of Key Largo, Florida, a distance of more than one thousand miles. The research project tested the effects of latency on the ability of a telesurgeon to perform effectively and identified the types of accommodations made by surgeons to surgical challenges. And very recently, a different team used a new smaller, lighter, and more portable robotic surgery system to perform simple surgery tasks assisted by the Penelope robot. Penelope responded to voice commands to provide and remove supplies to and from the surgical field, thus allowing a surgeon to simulate surgery robotically.

Today, technical issues must be resolved before the FDA would contemplate approval of telesurgery. A lot of bandwidth is needed to carry the images; transmission has to be fast, that is, when the surgeon actuates the controls; the response at the distant site needs to be essentially instantaneous with no latency; and the current "tremor" on the video screen needs to be eliminated. But these are technical issues that engineers and surgeons working together are in the process of resolving.

Putting It All Together

- Patient is Scanned in CAT or MRI
- Scan Sent to Simulator
- Surgeon "Practices" to Obtain Ideal
- Data Loaded Into Robot
- Robot Assists in Actual Surgery

It seems, therefore, that robotics will become as important in surgery as industrial robots have become to manufacturing. They can overcome certain obstacles or barriers, such as accessibility to certain tissues, distance (telesurgery), dexterity (the six degrees of freedom or a wristlike motion), and speed. They'll work only if robots become increasingly more intelligent and surgeons become highly skilled in their use. Surgeons, bioengineers, engineers, mathematicians, and information technology experts will need to come together. Many people think robotics will only become truly useful if they can also include some type of *haptics* (a sense of touch or feeling) feedback.

One can also imagine using the robot for a needle biopsy that is guided by an image. We previously discussed using needle biopsies for lesions seen on a mammogram. It can also be done with a robotic type of approach. This concept of image-guided, needle-based interventions with the robot can lead to less invasive approaches to obtaining a needed tissue diagnosis. As in the breast biopsy example, it can lead to faster recovery, less morbidity, fewer complications, and reduced costs. It will be increasingly used for biopsies of the prostate, biopsies of suspected metastases of cancer in the liver, and even for very delicate procedures, such as sampling the retina of the eye.

The surgical console used for robotic surgery will become the center of the surgeon's work world. There he or she will plan surgery, practice the complex portions of the case, direct the robot during the actual surgery, and study elements of the case afterward, just as the NFL teams study their weekend's efforts on Monday.

Since robots are basically information-driven surgical tools, the potential for the future of medicine is to transcend certain human limitations to increase consistency and quality. Hopefully, they can also promote better outcomes with lower costs.

MEGATRENDS IN SURGERY

Four major megatrends are occurring in relation to surgery and the operating room.

The first is that surgery is no longer needed for many diseases, where once it was a treatment mainstay. Duodenal ulcers are a good example of a disease now cured with antibiotics and treated with drugs to stop acid production. Surgery is rarely necessary anymore. Second, many procedures can be done in locations other than the operating room, like the various types of procedures done with interventional radiology, such as repairing an aortic aneurysm. Third, the OR has increasingly greater functionality. Witness the neuronavigational device and the many new types of imaging that assist the surgeon to be fully prepared for the patient's anatomy. Finally, the "new view" in the OR reveals image guidance as key to many surgical approaches, simulators to assist the trainee to become competent before working on a patient and to help the surgeon plan just the right surgery for the individual person. And the robot, to be preprogrammed for the case at hand, will increase functionality and reduce error.

THE MEGATRENDS
Operating Room of the Future

- ■ Fewer Procedures Will Need Surgery
- ■ Fewer Procedures Will Need OR
- ■ Extended Functionality of the OR
- ■ Room "With a New View"

Perhaps not a trend from the patient's perspective, but internists, traditionally considered "pill pushers," are using more and more invasive technologies with imaging assistance, and at the same time surgeons are using less invasive approaches in many circumstances. The two fields are converging more and more.

Simulation is a major transformational megatrend and is not just limited to the OR. I predict that all training in medical procedures will have a basis in simulation. Trainees will be required to demonstrate competence on the appropriate simulator before ever going near a live patient. This will be a fundamental change in how physicians (and also nurses and other health care providers) learn procedure-based medicine and it will then spill over into methods for didactic and conceptual learning as well.

WHAT YOU SHOULD KNOW

Given the profound changes coming into the operating room, such as new imaging techniques, simulation, robotics, and identification devices, it follows that more professionals, not fewer, will be needed in the operating room. This may sound counterintuitive, because isn't the reason to have all these new technologies, at least in part, to reduce the workload and hence the number of people required for the same procedure? In fact, surgeons, anesthesiologists, and nurses will need more training in technologies, computer expertise, and multitasking.

Implications of the Operating Room of the Future

- Need for More Professionals, Not Less
- Need for More Training and Expertise
- Surgery Designed for Specific Patient
- You Need to Ask Many Questions
    - Expertise of Surgeon?
    - Expertise of Hospital and Staff?
    - Need for Surgery vs Other Approach?
    - Open vs Laparoscopic Surgery?
    - Outpatient vs Inpatient Surgery?

Simulation for all these technologies will become ubiquitous, and nurses will increasingly be the preoperative and postoperative caregivers. With this level of technology, the operating room will be a place for the most highly educated, most highly trained, and the most experienced.

So return to our original scenario at the opening of this chapter, where I asked you to imagine having surgery in the year 2020. You will go through a scanner, such as a CAT scan or MRI, but one much more highly developed than today's equipment. The scan will be sent to the simulator where the surgeon literally practices the key aspects of the surgery and will be able to see your exact anatomy, even your own physiology down to a cellular and even a molecular level. The surgeon can practice to obtain the ideal approach to this surgical procedure and then load that data into the robotic assistant. The robot, still under the control of the surgeon will assist in the actual surgery—the surgery designed specifically for you. Another example of personalized medicine.

WHAT YOU CAN DO

Even today the changes in the OR are dramatic and rapid. You, as a patient or the loved one of a patient, need to know about these changes so that you can ask the surgeon, anesthesiologist, and nurses necessary questions. Ask first about the surgeon's expertise and experience in general and with the specific operation at hand. Ask how often this type of operation is done at the suggested hospital—in other words, is the staff experienced as well? Then ask about whether it can and will be done with a laparoscope or similar equipment—arthroscope, thoracoscope, and so forth. If not, why not? There may well be a very good reason, but you should know what it is.

Ask if this procedure can be done less invasively in the interventional radiology suite. Sometimes when the answer is no, it really relates to competition for cases, not whether it is technologically possible. Maybe it would mean that the surgeon loses control and hands you over to a radiologist for the procedure—and loses the fee in the process. This can be hard to discover, but you need to know. Does your surgeon use simulators to practice? And what about the residents or others who will assist the surgeon, do they have expertise, and do they have requirements to practice on simulators? These are just some of the questions that you need to ask in addition to the critical question of whether you really need the surgery at all.

Are there other approaches to dealing with the problem; if so, what are the pros and cons of each approach? You should also get a second opinion; ask your medical doctor who he or she recommends for this purpose. In the end, you will probably depend on your internist's and surgeon's expertise to guide you, but be sure to ask so that you can feel confident that you are going down the right path. Always remember in medicine, it's *your* body—and you are paying for the service.

CHAPTER 7

Your Medical Records—Digitized

If you've ever had to get a second opinion or go to a specialist, you will relate to this story. Susan Gerard always got her mammogram each year. She used her birthday as a reminder. Unfortunately, this time a mass was detected and she was sent for a biopsy. But it was *her* job to go pick up her mammogram and bring it to the hospital where the biopsy was to be performed. Bad news again, the biopsy was positive for cancer. So Susan was now sent to a major cancer center for consultation and treatment.

"Be sure to bring your mammogram, the surgeon's notes, and the pathology—not just the report but the actual slides from the laboratory."

So Susan, who was already stressed beyond belief, also had to worry about collecting all this stuff from all those places. Not easy. But specialists at a cancer center need complete information so that they can determine the best course of treatment. Simply stated, a better way of transmitting information, quickly and efficiently, is needed, without you, the patient, having to do it all. In effect, Susan became Federal Express; it should not be that way.

DIGITIZING MEDICAL INFORMATION

Medicine has always been about information—delivered, exchanged, and acted upon.

Data—from the symptoms and the physician's examination all the way to increasingly more complex test results—are combined with the best available medical knowledge to decide how to treat someone.

What's different now? The sources and quantity of information are increasing dramatically and this affects decisions. You may not yet have walked into an examining room and found your doctor sitting at a computer terminal or working with a personal digital assistant (PDA)—but you will soon. In the last decade, the laptop has replaced the microscope as the required piece of equipment for medical school students. In fact, the first week of medical school is now often called *boot camp*—for booting up your computer and learning to access information from the virtual library. As new generations of doctors fill the offices and hospitals, you will see how the use of the computer is growing as an integral part of medical practice. In this chapter, I will prepare you for what to expect when the computer takes on a much bigger role in medical information gathering and as a resource base for your care.

There is an old saying in medicine: you learn in relation to the patient you're treating right now. A doctor learns by studying about, for example, the patient with pneumonia in the office. Much more is learned at that time than by waiting to read a textbook or journal article on the living room sofa on Sunday afternoon. Today it sinks in; Sunday your doctor sinks in for a nap. Computers take this to a new level by enhancing the physician's ability to record and recall your data and quickly access information.

For example, you go to the doctor, who listens to your symptoms, checks you out, and decides penicillin is the best medication for your condition. The problem is that neither you nor your doctor remembers that a few years back, you had an allergic reaction to penicillin. It's somewhere in the doctor's paper chart, but that piece of information is not readily available. The computer, however, doesn't forget. Information retrieval is instantaneous and complete. As soon as the doctor enters the prescription into the computer, your allergy is flagged and you are spared the ordeal of finding out after the fact that you should not have taken that medication.

But there is more. The computer can help your physician choose a better treatment. Penicillin may not be the best medication in the first place for the infection that you have. The computer asks the physician what problem he or she is treating. The physician enters in *pneumonia*. The computer then says (putting aside the allergy question for now) that penicillin is not the best choice anymore for a pneumonia that develops at home and reports that the physician's infectious disease colleagues would suggest one of three antibiotics. The computer would also explain why penicillin is not as effective today and why choosing one of the other three antibiotics would be better.

And if a physician wishes to dig deeper, drop down menus take him or her in any number of directions, such as the usual causes of community-acquired pneumonia, the underlying conditions that may lead to pneumonia, the most commonly used antibiotics, and other aspects of therapy. Such on-the-spot updates will give doctors a much broader base of knowledge for making optimum decisions and they can learn while they work. So we can have both alerts (safety issues) and knowledge (education) built into the computer to assist us as caregivers.

So now your physician has determined what antibiotic to prescribe. Let's discuss prescriptions, those little sheets of paper written in hieroglyphics that you cannot understand. Soon, pharmacists won't decipher handwriting and you won't wait in line to drop it off at your pharmacy. Your doctor will send the prescription electronically to the pharmacist, quickly and accurately. If the pharmacist has a question it can be asked electronically.

In the future, each patient will have a Web location for his or her prescriptions and a password to gain access. The doctor will add your latest prescription to be filled, you will give the password to the pharmacist, and he or she will prepare the medication while also checking your other medications for possible drug-drug interactions that might be harmful. This will be helpful when you are traveling. Information is everywhere through the Internet. The amount of information being collected on a single patient is growing enormously.

Take CAT scans, which are increasingly used as a tool for diagnosis. A single scan on newer equipment can easily produce a thousand or more slices in seconds. It's simply not possible for the radiologist to look at a thousand pictures. So a whole new paradigm for analyzing images is needed. Throughout this chapter, I want to discuss with you the human factor in using technology—what to do when it is too much information and what you need to know when you sign on for testing or other diagnostic procedures.

My basic theme—and the key megatrend—is that all health care data needs to be digitized and in the not-too-distant future it will be. This will make for much better immediate care and, more important, for better continuity of care because the right information will be available at the right time to allow the right choices and decisions.

OPPORTUNITIES FROM DIGITIZING MEDICAL DATA

A host of opportunities will open before us, once medical information is digitized. Information now can be analyzed, organized, moved, viewed from different perspectives, and accessed and used by anyone who has privileges to the information.

What needs to be digitized? Well, it starts with the medical records that your physician and nurse keep with pen and paper today. This contains your history and physical exam information along with medication history, aller-gies, and a list of all past medical problems and the care plan for each of those that are active issues. But it also includes laboratory data, data from biopsies, all the information that comes from the various types of images, including X-rays and the information from medical monitors—blood pressure, pulse, respiration, and so on. And it includes your vaccination history from child-birth onward.

I mentioned some of this in the previous chapter while discussing the operating room of the future. The surgical team wants to have all of the nec-essary information readily available before surgery starts and throughout the case. But that information is scattered in many locations. The surgeon took notes in his or her office a few weeks ago and those are almost undoubtedly in a paper format. Someone from the anesthesiology department, likely a dif-ferent anesthesiologist from the one in the OR, saw and evaluated the patient, and those handwritten notes are needed, as are the X-rays, laboratory data, and the informed consent. Especially important is information about any past illnesses, such as heart disease or pulmonary disease, that could impact the surgical procedure and the postoperative care. All too often this information is simply not available to the surgeon and anesthesiologist at the time of sur-gery. It would be, if it was all electronic and digitized.

But this requires an infrastructure with standards and a vocabulary that is common across all of medicine. You know that doctors speak in a jargon all of their own, but you may not be aware that every specialty has its own jar-gon and abbreviations; it can even be hard for different physicians to under-stand each other. In any event, you as a patient need to have medical lingo converted into everyday usage. So until there is a standard infrastructure, stan-dard ways of inputting information, and a standard vocabulary, it will be dif-ficult for the digitized medical information to reach its full potential and be used by a primary care physician, specialist, surgeon, nurse, and yes, you, the patient, along with your family members.

What is digitized today and what is not? Most images, X-rays and the like, are now in digital format. Some X-rays like mammograms still tend to be in nondigital format, but this is changing as well. Most laboratory reports, such as blood counts, chemistries, and the like, are in digital format when they come from the laboratory. Much of the information on monitors in hospitals is in a digital format as well. The opportunity is there to bring all of that infor-mation together in the digital medical record.

But a lot of information is not yet digitized. Most biopsy reports are not, and equally important, your doctors' and nurses' notes tend to be handwritten on paper. Along with those are the pulse, blood pressure, and temperature results collected by your physician or nurse and likewise recorded in a handwritten format. But all this could be digitized. The issue is how much effort, how much change in provider productivity, and how much money it will cost to accomplish.

One standard that is being recommended today comes from the American Society for Testing and Materials (ASTM). They recommend a standard that will allow for flexible documents that will have the most important and timely information needed no matter where you might be. It would include your demographics (name, age, sex, identifiers), your insurance information, a list of all diagnoses, your medications and allergies, whatever care plan has been recommended, and any other special information.

The idea is that if just this much information were available, no matter where you were, it could be useful, if not lifesaving. By keeping the amount of data manageable, it can and therefore will be collected readily and made available for your needs. Make the list too long or too complex and it will never get done, and hence becomes a useless concept. It is similar to the "80-20 rule"—you can have 80 percent of what you need with 20 percent of the effort needed to get all of it.

Digitizing Medical Data

- History and Physical Examination
- Past Medical History
  —Other Illnesses
  — Medications
- Laboratory Results
- Images
- Blood Pressure, Pulse (from monitors)

The advantage of a digital medical record is easily available information, any time and any place. It offers the opportunity to intercept errors and to monitor patients from a distance. It can improve quality by giving prompts or alerts to clinicians. For example, just as your e-mail program on your computer may pop up a message to tell you that you have an e-mail waiting, electronic medical records alert your physician, so that he or she will know to look for an abnormal lab result or an abnormal chest X-ray report or to adjust a drug dosage.

Similarly, the electronic medical record can notify the patient of an impending problem. For example, most people with diabetes check their blood sugar a number of times a day. These measurements could be digitized and placed into your medical record with an automatic notification coming back to you—and to your physician—if the sugar readings are tending to be too high or too low.

Some interesting studies going on now involve individuals who have congestive heart failure. They keep a digital bathroom scale and weigh themselves every day. The information is automatically sent to their care manager, and if a person's weight is going up over a few days, it may indicate a need for a medication change. The point is that this can be picked up long before the patient starts to feel short of breath or has other symptoms of worsening heart failure. It can prevent visits to the doctor or to the emergency room and, most importantly, can reduce the frequency of hospitalizations—and reduce costs. Now that is a real advance.

HURDLES TO OVERCOME

There are a lot of problems today. Medical information is essentially locked up where it cannot be easily accessed and cannot be analyzed. Frequent information handlers are another problem. In the hospital, when a doctor goes off duty, he or she usually gives a report to the doctor who is covering overnight or for the weekend. But the more information is exchanged, the more opportunity there is for it to be lost or changed.

Remember the old telephone game where you whisper a few words in one person's ear and that person turns to the person on the other side and whispers in his ear and it goes around a circle of five or seven people and by the time it gets back to you the message has been totally changed? That happens today in medicine all the time. Information gets diluted; meaning becomes lost. Digitized data on the other hand, unless it's manipulated, retains its original context. Information can be shared quickly and with multiple people at the same time.

These problems need to be solved—today. But I predict that they won't be solved unless some type of incentive is created to assist in the transition. Frankly, it's a major problem for medicine today. Let's look back on the story of Susan Gerard at the beginning of this chapter. In my opinion, it's something of a crime that she is the one who had to do all the data collection in order to get her medical information to all the right caregivers. There are other problems of a similar nature that occur all too often today. Medical students are frequently asked to serve as runners to go to the laboratory each afternoon and pick up information on the patients for the ward in which they're serving.

Often, the surgical resident gets the job of going down to X-ray and bringing the patient's films up to the operating room in preparation for surgery. The medical resident looks up all the information about his or her patients and writes it all down on an index card before the attending physician arrives for rounds. And the doctor who is being signed out to by another physician is, hopefully, writing down all the pertinent information about each patient so that it will be available if a problem occurs during the weekend or evening.

What a waste of time and effort, not to mention an enormous amount of duplication. This is simply not the way that medical information should be transferred from person to person. It's changing, but it's changing at a snail's pace. There is a motivation, of course, and that motivation is to get at medicine's capabilities to access and analyze information. But when an electronic medical record is introduced into a physician's office practice or into a hospital setting, in general, physician productivity tends to go down for a substantial period of time. From the physician's perspective, it is taking more time to get the same job done, and the physician tends not to appreciate the longer-term benefit that having the information digitized will ultimately create. Particularly important are the enhancements to patient safety and quality of care for all the reasons discussed in the patient safety chapter, but the physician is in a time crunch today and not focusing on the future.

Today only about 18 percent of hospitals have some type of relatively complete electronic medical record. Perhaps 25 percent of large group physician practices have electronic medical records, but certainly less than 10 percent of smaller practices have them. There is a long way to go.

What are some of the innovations that are being built into the electronic medical record? I have mentioned electronic prescribing already and in the hospital we sometimes call this *computer physician order entry* (CPOE). I describe it in more detail in the chapter on patient safety, but in its simplest format, the physician goes to the computer, enters his or her password, looks up a patient and then enters the drug order. The computer will alert the physician if there is an allergy to that drug, if the patient is taking other drugs that might have an adverse interaction, or if there is a need to adjust the dosage because of kidney disease.

All this can be done on the office computer, on a PDA, and wirelessly from any location at any time. The electronic prescription can be sent directly to the pharmacy and the physician can be alerted if the patient does not pick up the medications within a certain time frame. Dr. John Halamka at Beth Israel Deaconess Hospital in Boston noted they have about two million ambulatory visits per year.[1] Evidence there suggests that adverse drug events occurred somewhere between 1 percent and 7 percent of the time among patients who were given a prescription. Each of these events costs between two- to five-thousand dollars in extra clinic visits, possibly an emergency room visit, or even a hospitalization.

Let's assume that their electronic prescribing system decreases adverse drug events by 50 percent. This would mean that, at the lowest end, a 1 percent rate drops to a 0.05 percent rate. This may not seem like a lot, but if it's spread over those who got a prescription among the two million visits, then it's a significant reduction in adverse events. Computer order entry will stop the handwriting errors, the dosage errors, the drug-drug interaction problems, and will pick up the known allergies. That is a real advance.

Computer order entry also has the opportunity for decision support systems not only with built-in alerts but also with built-in knowledge to inform and teach the provider on the spot. Patient tracking and verification can also be included so the physician can know that the patient actually picked up the medication.

With all these advantages, why is it taking so long for the creation of electronic medical records? The banking industry and the financial services industry of Wall Street have been effectively using digitized information for years. But it's important to remember that the data from the bank or from Wall Street is generally numeric in origin and fairly simple to organize. Computers are excellent at analyzing this sort of numeric data. But clinical information is inherently more complex; it is more important, and it's critical that it be correct. Clinical information today is for the most part not in a digitized format, and only some of it such as laboratory data is numeric to start. It becomes a complicated, expensive problem to resolve.

Remember that we have to include digitized images—remember those thousand slices from the CAT scan of the chest—and we have to put the information into a contextual format. You have watched your physician write out a prescription, but even the medication order is rather complex. Taking

100 milligrams of a medicine three times a day sounds simple. But we do have to include the possibility of drug-drug interactions, dosage ranges based on age or illness, and alerts for appropriate uses.

The rules are different in different circumstances. The information that is important for a surgeon to know before prescribing a painkiller after surgery is much different from the information for a medical oncologist working with complicated and toxic drugs. The information that is necessary for an internist to take good care of a diabetic patient also is substantially different. The medications for a five-month-old girl would have one set of rules, but a much different set is needed for a ninety-five-year-old woman. The same medication given to a pregnant woman requires a different set of rules from an adult male of the same age. This is a lot different from when a stock analyst compares one company with another; the rules are pretty much the same from company to company and stock to stock.

Another big problem in creating an electronic medical record is that the clinical data is usually not all in the same place. Today it is in one or more doctor's offices, one or more hospitals, multiple laboratories and radiology offices, perhaps at a physical therapy site, or at an emergency room. So it all needs to find a way to come together.

There is yet another issue. A clerk in the bank works for the bank and the bank can say, "Look, this is the way we keep our information," and the teller will keep the information in that fashion. Physicians tend to be independent. They don't work for the hospital, and if using the electronic system slows them down, they avoid using it. This is what I mean by saying that the incentives are different and that there has not been much incentive within medicine to drive the process ahead.

Usually the only incentive in a hospital or a large physician practice is to reduce costs as a result of the new information system. But collecting clinical information into an electronic medical record is not really about costs—although it can reduce them—but about better medical care. But that is hard to quantify in dollar terms, so hospitals are loath to spend the extra dollars to help the physician or nurse learn how to use the system efficiently.

All of this has been made worse by the lack of standards and infrastructure. Each vendor of electronic medical records has its own proprietary system. There is no recognized authority requiring open architecture of the software, ease of use, or interoperability. In short, there needs to be adjudication of standards. This is like the railroads in the 1850s. Every railroad had its own track gauge, the distance between the tracks, so a freight car could not be moved from one railroad to the other. The cargo had to be unloaded and then reloaded on to the other railroad's freight car. Passenger trains had the same problem. Eventually the railroads realized that this was a problem for their customers and that they had to solve it. They agreed on a single track gauge. It was the railroad companies that also established our current system of standard time across the country. This allowed for schedules that anyone could follow from coast to coast. We need this type of agreement on standards in medical records.

A number of large companies have been producing their versions of electronic medical record systems. These companies have invested an enormous amount of time, people, and dollars to make these systems as robust as possible. One of the problems is that computer software writers are generally not clinically trained, so they do not think like clinicians, they do not understand the work of clinicians, and they do not understand the style of practice.

Why Digitize?

- ■ All Data Available
- ■ Access Anytime, Anyplace
- ■ Reduce Handoff Errors, Information Dilution
- ■ Create Digital Hospital
- ■ Create Computer-Integrated Medicine
- ■ Distance Medicine
  - — You Access Provider
  - — Provider Accesses You
- ■ Data Mining

For example, consider how an internist might make rounds in the hospital. He goes from patient to patient as the first stop in the morning. When finished, he may then go to radiology to confer with the radiologists on specific X-rays that were taken yesterday. Then it's on to the laboratory to see pathology specimens, then a stop to consult with a colleague. All the while, the physician is getting phone calls about this patient or that result. In short, it is a very discontinuous type of workflow. An electronic medical record to suit the needs of the physician would have to be designed with this type of discontinuous workflow in mind.

Paper records work well for physicians, because over time they have created a system that is both efficient and effective. I am on the board of a company, Salar Inc., that is trying to solve a portion of this problem. In designing their software, the leaders spent many hours in meetings with physicians to learn what they needed and wanted. One thing that was important was for the screen to look like what the doctors use today with paper.

In other words, "Don't try to change how we work, but rather honor how we work with how you put together your software." So far, physician acceptance and response has been positive as a result of this approach.

Physicians complain, often frequently and sometimes even vividly, that the systems they are using are not as robust as they should be. When you turn on your computer to write a letter, the program responds quickly and effectively. But the software for the current electronic medical records often seems to be slow, and the hardware is not as powerful as it might be. The vendors appear to sell now and innovate later with upgrades of significance being slow to emerge. I don't want to be overly critical; they are doing their best in a competitive marketplace. But more needs to be done.

I don't use the software program Quicken, but people who do tell me that this is a system that creates "positive emotion." It works in an intuitive manner; it follows the way that a person uses their checkbook and as a result, the learning curve is greatly reduced. Not so for most electronic medical records. They are slow and cumbersome and physicians get frustrated and impatient. But changes are coming. These large vendors are appreciating that they need to satisfy the physicians if indeed their systems are going to be sold and used.

One approach is to have a system to customize what the doctor "sees," while still using the common underlying architecture. For example, a cardiac surgeon needs to "see" only certain information and likes to have that presented in a fashion that is quite different from, for example, the cardiologist or the internist who each have a different set of needs, a different mode of practice. So companies are creating "intelligent filters" so they can design from the clinician's perspective.

THE INTERNET, MEDICAL RECORDS, AND MEDICAL INFORMATION

What about the Internet? At its most basic, the Internet is the pipeline through which data can be moved. As a patient moves about, whether that is across town, across the country, or across the planet, the information potentially can be readily available through the Internet.

Ultimately, this will transform medicine—with records available anywhere, anytime, instantly. But the Internet is more than just a pipeline; it is a source of information. It is a location where one can go for disease guidance, access to support groups, and in so doing can create a more informed patient, a more informed population, and a more informed health care provider. But the user must be able to differentiate the useful from the junk, of which there is much. (Suggestion: When looking up health information, go to sites that are reputable, like major hospitals or medical schools. Another option is to use HON or Health on the Net (www.hon.ch), a not-for-profit Swiss foundation operating out of Geneva, which is a portal to medical information on the Internet.)

Through the Internet, the physician or hospital can get information to a patient in advance of a visit so that the patient arrives better informed and with any needed information. As I suggested earlier, the Internet serves as a method for a physician to maintain a watchful eye on how a patient is doing by using digital scales, digital blood pressure machines, or digital glucose monitoring. Mostly, this is still in the talk stage, but I predict we will be seeing quite a bit of it within less than five years.

I also predict that we will see the "googlization" of medical information. A big issue for a physician is the need to find certain data, quickly, from the mountain of information that has been collected. At best this can be time-consuming, and at worst it might not yield what is needed. I can think of multiple times when I was asked to see a patient who had, literally, a chart that was three to four inches thick and sometimes even multiple charts of that thickness. Trying to hunt through them to find relevant information for a consultation was a timely chore.

Hurdles to Success

- Lack of Standards
  No Common Vocabulary
  No Common Infrastructure
  No "Force" to Create/Insist on Standards
- Software Not Created by Clinicians
- Software/Hardware Not Adequately Robust
- Software Not Intuitive (Reduces productivity, at least at first)

So why did I say "googlization"? Well, because Google's core competency is search algorithms. This competency can be harnessed to search the medical record for the relevant data freeing the clinician from thumbing through the entire chart and all the stuff that will accumulate throughout one's lifetime of medical care. But again, this can only be done if the information has been digitized from the start.

This is one approach to make data more readily useful to the practitioner. I have also suggested that filters to select what is needed by a specific practitioner can be useful. In the OR a mountain of information is generated during the course of the surgery. In order to maintain situational awareness, the surgeon, anesthesiologist, and nurse need to have that information centralized and reduced to its essence.

For example, some companies are coming together and working with Massachusetts General Hospital and Memorial Sloan Kettering Cancer Center to develop a single monitor in the operating room that will show all the relevant and critical data—and only that data. The practitioners will not need to look all around the room at various monitors and equipment to see what is going on, but rather be able to see in one location in clear view the most important information.

PRIVACY

We do need to talk about privacy, which is a critical issue. If your medical information gets to the wrong person, whom I will for this purpose label as a *bad person,* it could be to your disadvantage. Perhaps it will mean that you cannot get insurance. Perhaps it means that it will restrict your ability to get employment. Or it may mean that someone, having found out that you are, for example, diabetic, will bombard you with e-mails selling drugs, insulin, and so forth. So privacy is critical and how protecting privacy is accomplished in the future is going to be important.

In the past, your medical record was kept by your physician in your physician's office or in the hospital record in the hospital record room. Pretty much no one else had access to that information. If digitized and not properly secured, then others can gain access to it. If you are a victim of identity theft, will the thief be able to use that data to access your medical records, or will only you have a pass code? One of the big issues is to assure that your data remains private and can be accessed only by the appropriate individuals and only with your consent.

YOUR MEDICAL RECORD

This brings me to an important point and it is sort of a paradigm shift in the way we all need to think about medical records. First of all, the information collected really is *your* medical record.

It is not the hospital's or the doctor's. As the owner of the data, you need a method to access it yourself and to make it available to any doctor or hospital of your choosing, no matter where you may be at the time. With digitized medical records, this can become a reality. Today I venture to say that you do not know whether or not you had a tetanus shot within the last ten years. If you step on a nail and go to the emergency room, you will be asked this question and since you cannot remember, you will be given a tetanus shot just to be on the safe side.

If you go to a specialist at the referral of your internist and the specialist does not have access to the CAT scan that was taken two weeks ago, he may simply send you down the hall for another one, because sometimes that is simpler than trying to get the old information.

The concept of the personal health record is important. Each of us needs to have a mechanism whereby we, as well as our health care providers, can access that information in a simple rapid fashion, while at the same time protecting our privacy. Today, in Iraq, more than eighteen thousand soldiers are wearing a new type of dog tag. The *personal information carrier* (PIC) is preloaded with an individual's demographics, including medical data such as allergies, medication, blood type, and so on. The future plan for the military is to include a baseline CT scan on the digital dog tag as well.

Internet

■ Internet is a "Pipe" – Information Flow
■ Source of Information for
  Disease Guidelines
  Disease Explainations
  Support Groups
  Quackery (or at least bad information)
■ Telemedicine/ Distance Medicine
■ "Googlization" of Medical Data

If a soldier was wounded in the field, the old system called for a medic to fill out a simple cardboard form that included a stick figure drawing. The medic could mark where a wound was and make another mark where a tourniquet was applied. The medic might indicate that he gave a medication, such as penicillin, by noting a large P on the card and a large M for morphine. Today the medic writes all that out, not on a piece of cardboard, but on a PDA. The digital dog tag is inserted into the PDA, which uploads the information. The soldier is taken to the back field hospital, where the next level of caregiver inserts the PIC into a computer and downloads that information.

If additional medical care is given, it is recorded on the computer and from there onto the PIC. The PIC, which now has all the medical information, goes with the soldier to the major hospital in Germany where additional medical care is given, and the PIC is again updated. The soldier is airlifted to the United States, say, to Walter Reed Army Medical Center, still wearing the dog tag with all the information about everything that's been done.

The early PICs were capable of 64 MB (megabytes). New ones can hold 2 GB (gigabytes), which is enough capacity to hold CAT scan information, MRIs, and more. Not only that, the newer PICs have wireless capability, which means that there is no need to insert the dog tag into the PDA or the computer; the data is just uploaded and downloaded quickly and effortlessly.

The military is working on a concept called the *holographic medical electronic record* (HoLoMER). The idea is to include not just basic medical information, but also the digitized CT scan and much more, such as the soldier's electrocardiogram and blood chemistries. In time, it will include a 3-D body scan that can include not just anatomic information, but also functional and physiologic information of the sort discussed in the imaging chapter. This total body information will then be instantly available when a soldier is injured, wounded, or develops an illness, now or much later in life. You can expect that this approach will become commonplace in the civilian sector in the not-too-distant future as well.

My personal belief is that all of us need to have some sort of PIC equivalent that we keep in our pocket. It might be like a credit card that has a built-in chip that can store this type of information. Think of what happened in Hurricane Katrina. People left the city, and many needed medical care, but their medical information was buried under eight feet of water. If you had your own medical information, say, on a card in your wallet, chances are you would have taken it with you when you fled New Orleans. Personally, I think there is something reassuring about having your personal medical information with you at all times.

But there are other approaches. One is called the National Health Information Network. A few years ago President George W. Bush said in his State of the Union address that health records should become electronic within a decade. He then appointed a physician to head the Office of National Coordinator for this network concept. The basic idea is that all health information should be digitized. Then no matter where it resides, be it your doctor's office, a hospital, an emergency room, a laboratory, or a radiology office, it could all be accessed quickly and effortlessly through the Internet.

Perhaps you are visiting a relative out of state and you need to go the emergency room. You would simply give your identification number and that could call up the information, but it could be accessed only with a password. Although, you might allow certain critical information to be accessible without a password, in case you were unconscious or unable to communicate.

Probably the system will be set up on a region-by-region basis to start. But the basic problems we discussed need to be resolved, such as getting various systems to interact together through an open architecture or having required interfaces so that all systems can "plug and play" together. It will probably require a national identification card, but this is of concern to some civil libertarians among others, and it is not certain how or whether a national ID card will be created. Certainly there are the same privacy concerns.

You might think it would be hard to surreptitiously access the information, but here is an example of how it can happen. A contract was given to a specific vendor to maintain medical data on the military. As told to me, that same vendor had some business in China, and the two elements were run on some of the same computers. Suddenly it was realized that the Chinese government had been able to access the medical information, not only of the military, but also of senior members of the executive branch. So much for security and privacy!

Perhaps the national system of automated and linked ATMs could be co-opted to carry medical information as well. Banks have worked out security systems and password systems, and in general, these work quite well. But it is clear that the information about you is fundamentally your property. Not everyone agrees with this concept yet. Physicians think of the records in their office as *their* records, and most hospitals and other health care providers act in the same fashion. But this will change—because it must.

Another change will be the ability of the health care provider community to access you—to give you medical information that can be helpful to you and your care. This can improve quality by reversing the basic process. You as a patient can be sent alerts and updates.

The diabetic patient can be notified that blood sugar has been running high. The patient who wants to stop smoking can be sent regular updates of smoking cessation approaches, and the individual who is trying to lose weight can be sent reminders, prods, and useful suggestions on a regular basis. Setting this up with proper algorithms should be relatively trivial.

Accessing your own medical record will be a change—for the doctor, the hospital, and the patient. But it will come. Some decisions will need to be made, however. Should you get your data before the doctor has had time to discuss it with you? Say you had a biopsy that showed cancer. The pathologist places this information in the electronic medical record; you see it and naturally become anxious. Probably better that there be a delay—but only a slight delay—so that your personal physician can give you this news and concurrently discuss what the next steps will be to deal with it.

COMPUTER INTEGRATION OF MEDICAL CARE

A possibly grander scheme is to convert today's hospital into, basically, a computer-integrated facility, and as a result, medicine into the computer integration of medical care. Such shifts require hospitals to totally rethink themselves. The grand challenge is for the hospital information system to be able to integrate everything known about a patient. This information should be used and useful to manage the patient's care. It can go further in accessing the supply chain or anything else relevant to the patient's care. Then the information can be maintained to give indicators of care and safety monitors.

The information can be mined for statistical process control, just like an industry. There can be outcome indicators in real time and the information from these outcome indicators can be related back to individual patients within an overall patient population with a given problem. But all this will require that the hospital reconsider how it organizes its departments, its logistics, and its finances. It will require breaking down the stovepipes or the silos that are inherent in the way medicine is practiced today.

We can go even further and consider that the computer integration of medical care will include the representation of all that is known today about the patient and tie it to all that is known about biology and medicine. These are two massive visions, but they can be done in pieces, and what is exciting is that much of it can be done now, once medical information has been digitized and is accessible.

DISTANCE MEDICINE

Let's talk a bit about distance medicine, a somewhat broader concept than telesurgery. The concept is that anyone—the world's expert—can see a patient through *telemedicine,* can see the patient's X-rays and the pathology specimen. This brings the expert to the patient, rather than the other way around. Telemedicine can offer consultation services to rural or underserved communities without the need to fly in the expert.

In Idaho a program has been started recently that allows the obstetrician and pediatrician in a remote hospital to call in to a large medical center when a premature baby is born. The plan is to transfer the baby to the medical center's neonatal intensive care unit, but that may take a few hours to accomplish. Telemedicine allows the neonatologist to see, actually examine, and consult on the baby. The neonatologist can use the electronic stethoscope to listen to the heart and lungs and abdomen. He or she can see the electrocardiogram and the X-rays that have been taken and can teleconference with the local physicians and the parents. This means that definitive care can begin sooner. It also means that the parents meet the neonatologist and have begun a relationship with him or her before they ever reach that very scary medical center. This helps relieve anxiety at a time of great stress and also helps the neonatologist to obtain a full medical history before the baby and the parents arrive.

Following is another example of planning treatment from a distance. Some types of strokes will benefit from the clot-busting drug tPA. But some patients would be harmed by receiving this drug, so the standard of care is to get a patient to a center that treats a lot of strokes, obtain a CAT scan to determine the type of stroke, and then administer the tPA if it is appropriate. But here's the rub, tPA only works if it can be given in the first few hours after the onset of the stroke. The result is that relatively few patients actually ever get tPA.

Mostly this is because they get to care too late for it to be effective. Only about 1 percent of stroke patients overall get tPA, yet it can be an exceptionally valuable treatment. Imagine for a moment a patient who comes into the emergency room paralyzed on one side and having difficulty speaking. The CAT scan, done right across the hall from the ER, demonstrates that the type of stroke is the right type and the tPA is given. Forty-five minutes later, the patient is sitting up on the edge of the gurney moving both arms and legs and speaking normally. I can tell you it is one of the most remarkable and nearly miraculous things that a physician can witness, and of course, for the patient and the patient's family, it is almost beyond belief.

The point is that telemedicine can make this type of information available before the patient gets to a major medical center, and this may allow the early start of tPA. It might work like this. The ambulance has a camera, so the patient can be virtually examined by the physician at the major medical center. And there is a miniaturized CT scanner onboard the ambulance. The scan can be done, read by the stroke expert via telemedicine technologies, and the tPA started while still en route. This could have a truly dramatic impact on the consequences of a stroke. Work is under way to create these miniaturized CT scanners. A few years from now, this could be a reality.

Here is yet another use of distance medicine. Today's intensive care unit is filled with very sick patients with complicated problems. More often than not, intensivists do not staff these units around the clock, seven days a week. In part, this is simply because not enough trained intensivists are available, because hospitals find it too expensive to hire the additional physicians, and because tradition and culture dictate that the individual physician remain in control of his or her own patient. But it is clear that having the intensivist available can make a significant difference in patient outcomes.

A company named Visicu has created the ability to monitor multiple patients in multiple ICUs from a distance. Doctors Michael Breslow and Brian Rosenfeld began their studies at Johns Hopkins Bayview Hospital in Baltimore and later founded the company. Visicu has found that a single physician can monitor fifty or more patients. In each room, a camera is trained on the patient that can be focused in and out to get close-up shots for the intensivist from the computer. The intensivist can also see the information from the monitors, such as blood pressure, pulse, and respirations, and also have access to the laboratory data, medication lists, and so on.

They can set up certain alerts that will direct the intensivist's attention to a given patient. Then based on what they see and hear and based on additional information that they may request from the nurse, the intensivist can order changes in medication or fluids, X-rays, or other procedures. This system works, and it has been shown to reduce mortality, reduce the length of stay in the intensive care unit, and generally improve care. Think of how this approach could have a major impact on the care of outpatients as well. The Visicu approach could be used to monitor patients at home with complex diseases, such as the combination of diabetes and heart failure. So instead of monitoring a few thousand ICU patients, the same technology could be used to monitor many hundreds of thousands of patients who need ongoing attentive care.

DIGITAL HOSPITAL

Digitization is not just about medical records; the concept is a digital hospital or digital medicine. An individual that I know developed a *cardiac arrhythmia*—an irregularity of the heart rhythm that was causing him some discomfort and concern. He was sent to a top cardiologist at an outstanding medical center where he had a procedure called *electro physiology* done to correct the problem.

Basically, it involved inserting a catheter into the artery in the groin and passing it up through the aorta into the heart and then finding the site in the heart from where the abnormal rhythm was developing. That site was cauterized so that it will no longer produce the abnormal rhythm—a terrific technology that is discussed in the chapter on devices.

Everything seemed to go fine, and my friend was kept overnight in the hospital for observation. He was awakened the next morning at 5:30 to have his vital signs taken and breakfast was brought in at 7:00 a.m. It was Saturday and by 10:30 that morning, the physician had not come in to discuss the procedure or the results, and there was no word as to whether the physician was scheduled to make rounds that Saturday anyway. So my friend signed himself out. The charge nurse insisted that he was leaving against medical advice, but he saw no reason to stay if his physician was not going to come by to review the results of the procedure.

This meant, unfortunately, that he left the hospital without the knowledge of what had been completed, was disappointed—indeed angry—that there had been no discussion, and had to wait until Monday to contact the physician to have the discussion that should have occurred on Saturday. On the other hand, the physician probably had a long week and felt he did not need to go into the hospital since a discussion could certainly wait until Monday. Personally, I think the physician forgot that everything may have seemed just fine to him, but that when you are the patient it is hard to be *patient* and wait a few days to get the results.

A concept called *Mr. Rounder* could have made this whole problem go away. I learned about it from Dr. Peter Gross, chairman of medicine at Hackensack University Medical Center in New Jersey. Basically, Mr. Rounder is a two-way video/audio device that allows a physician to visit a patient in the hospital from a distance. It is a cart carrying a monitor that allows the patient to see the physician, and just above the monitor is a camera that relays a picture of the patient back to the physician.

The doctor is sitting at his computer, which in turn has a camera mounted above the monitor taking a picture of the physician. So doctor and patient can see and talk to each other. But there is more to it than that. The physician can control the movement of this cart with a joystick and literally wheel it from hospital room to room. It can be dressed up a little bit to make it sort of fun. Instead of just looking like a cart with a monitor on it, it can sport a white coat and the monitor can represent the physician's face. Hence the name Dr. Rounder—a built-in two-way video teleconferencing ability. Patients like it as do the physicians. By the way, it can be used not only for the physician to interact with the patient, but also for the physician to interact with the nurse or to have a consult with another physician.

My friend would have benefited had this system been in place. His physician could have been at home and taken just the few minutes necessary to send Dr. Rounder to the bedside, where the two of them could have discussed the results of his procedure. It would have saved a lot of grief. The doctor could stay away, but still allow the patient to go home with a full understanding of what had been done.

"Dr. Rounder"

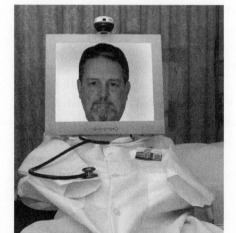

Courtesy Thomas Jemski, University of Maryland School of Medicine.

For the physician or nurse in the hospital, having a computer at the nurse's desk is not really convenient. When you are with a patient you would like to be able to quickly look up some information without trudging back down the hall to the nurse's station. Hence the concept of the *computer on wheels* (COW), which is basically a computer on a mobile cart with a battery that is wirelessly connected to an electronic medical record and allows the physician or nurse to move the computer to the bedside while interacting with the patient.

One can directly enter vital signs and other data about the patient, and it can also be useful in the operating room, as it can move with the patient as the patient goes from the operating room to the recovery room and into a regular bed later. When the computer on wheels was first installed on the coronary care unit of the hospital where I was CEO, the residents found that it cut their workday by nearly an hour. This was in part because they no longer needed to come in early to look up laboratory and other data, write it down on a card, and then be prepared for their rounds with their attending physician.

Instead, they brought the COW with them on work rounds and could look up information on the spot. Actually, they found it was efficient to bring two COWS on rounds. One was for looking up written data and the other for accessing the digitized X-rays. It also increased safety because it eliminated the opportunity for writing down incorrect data—a frequent cause of error in medical situations.

Instead of a COW, how about using a PDA? PDAs are too small to look at some pieces of information, and you can only see so much on the screen at one time. But they can be carried in your pocket, and with wireless technology, it is possible to access information, see and adjust medications, and write an order for additional testing. If the physician is in the cafeteria having lunch when his beeper beeps, he can use his cell phone to call back to the floor nurse who paged him and find out what the problem is. Then, after checking the patient's medical record via his PDA, he can write a new prescription, all the while still remaining in the cafeteria. So he was able to finish lunch, the nurse on the unit got the problem addressed promptly, and most important, the patient benefited from immediate action.

The digital hospital will have RFID (radio frequency identification) technology that tracks where every patient, doctor, staff member, and piece of equipment is at any time. This means that a physical therapist will not go to Mrs. Jones's room now, because the computer says she is off to radiology. It will mean greatly increased efficiency, greatly improved morale of staff (because of less wasted time), and greatly improved care with enhanced safety.

Patients will have a touch screen in their room where they can order their own food from a menu built around their own needs (low salt, etc.) and will be able to interact with the nurse directly. They will also be able to call up education programs on the procedure they are scheduled to have and review the potential side effects of their medications. And all the medications will be bar coded for safety and for tracking their utilization.

It also means that the hospital personnel—and you, for that matter—will know that the ICU has a problem with antibiotic resistant staph, that community acquired pneumococcal pneumonia does or does not tend to be resistant to penicillin, and whether the *E. coli* in urinary tract infections are likely to be resistant to the most commonly used antibiotics. This will give everyone an advantage in promptly treating infections with the best antibiotic or engaging in the needed protective measures to reduce spread of the resistant staph in the ICU.

MEDICAL EDUCATION AND SIMULATION

I wrote about using simulation for teaching medical procedures such as inserting a chest tube, performing endoscopy or training for laparoscopic surgery. Simulators in the years to come will totally change the way health care providers are trained in procedure-based skills. What about cognitive skills—clinical judgment? The technologies are not as far along here but I predict that the digitization of medical information will allow skill development here as well. Dr Bruce Jarrell and his colleagues at the University of Maryland Medical School have developed prototypes of systems that both train and measure clinical judgment as the student progresses. Systems like this will fundamentally change medical education going into the future. And, like their procedural counterpart simulators, they will test the student's competence—the key to allowing advancement to the next level of clinical responsibility.

DATA MINING

With data increasingly available in digitized form, it will become possible to data mine. Of course, removing identifying information will be a critical first step to maintaining privacy. Already some examples of data mining have proven to be useful and successful. All drugs have side effects. The issue is always to decide if the benefits outweigh the risks.

Premature infants sometimes develop a severe infection called sepsis. Antibiotics are absolutely essential, but what is the best regimen? A combination of two drugs, ampicillin and gentamicin, has been the standard for many years. But gentamicin can cause hearing loss and kidney problems if the blood levels get too high. As a result it is important to check the blood levels and make dosage adjustments as necessary. This is certainly doable, but it adds complexity to the care.

Some neonatologists started to use ampicillin plus another drug called cefotaxime. Cefotaxime is also a broad spectrum antibiotic, but it has less toxic potential than gentamicin, and blood levels need not be obtained; as a result, many pediatric intensivists prefer this combination. But which combination is really better? No one really knew, but everyone had his or her opinion.

A large hospital system with multiple neonatal intensive care units has been able to keep the information in a digitized format over a number of years. They were able to mine the data of all the premature infants who developed sepsis at each of their hospitals and demonstrated that the older, albeit more potentially toxic regimen that included gentamicin, was better—fewer babies died of sepsis. This is the sort of information that has not been readily available in the past, and this type of analysis is relatively easy to do, is inexpensive, and can greatly help in weighing approaches to medical care.

It depends on having the information digitized from the start. Think of the controversy over Vioxx, the pain- and inflammation-reducing drug from Merck. The fact that Vioxx was associated with a slightly increased frequency of heart attacks was not apparent in the early studies of the drug. It was recognized only when a large study was initiated that sought to determine if Vioxx would also be helpful in reducing the frequency of polyps in the colon and hence reducing colon cancer.

The increased heart attack risk could have been learned earlier if the information on every patient prescribed Vioxx was part of the national health information database as a result of the electronic medical record. Then it would have been easy and inexpensive to mine the data to determine if in fact there was an association between use of Vioxx and increased frequency of heart attacks—or any other problem. By the way, the trial regarding polyps was discontinued early when Vioxx was withdrawn from the market, but the results are in: Vioxx does indeed reduce the onset of polyps.

Actually, the opportunities for useful medical research with digitized information are huge. If you can access data, then you can do epidemiologic research, public health research, and administrative research. By the latter, I am thinking of things such as cost analysis. A new drug might be more expensive, and hence, on first blush, the thought is that it should not be used. But if the drug should prove to be superior and an individual requires less medical attention, fewer hospitalizations, or fewer emergency room admissions, then the added expense for the drug becomes quite acceptable.

Data mining can prove very valuable. These broad population-based studies will become relevant—and quickly—for the individual person who needs a drug, a procedure, or advice on lifestyle modification.

WHY DIGITIZATION IS SO IMPORTANT

Let me end this chapter with another story somewhat like the one with which I began. A gentleman I have known for many years developed something called an *acoustic neuroma*. Basically, this is a tumor that develops from the nerve that runs from the brain to the ear. It tends to develop in the narrow canal in which the nerve passes through the skull. This is the same canal that the facial nerve passes through on its way to control the muscles of the face.

As you can probably imagine, a small tumor growing in an equally small bony canal puts pressure on one or both of these nerves and ultimately causes symptoms like dizziness, pain, or muscle weakness in the face. Treatment takes a number of approaches. One is surgery, and several others use radiation therapy. It will suffice for the purpose of my story to say that controversies abound as to which procedure is the better procedure and in fact it probably depends in part on the patient's situation, but it also depends in part on the physician's expertise. Certainly, it is essential to have a highly experienced well-trained physician; the treatment options here are not for amateurs.

So he was trying to determine what the best option was, and that meant visiting a number of experienced surgeons and radiation therapists and getting their evaluation and recommendations. But that meant getting his CAT scan, MRI, and other information to each of the various specialists and then getting their reports sent back to his primary physician. Sometimes it took not days but literally months, and the patient eventually resorted to having the reports faxed to his own home so that he could hand-deliver them back to his primary physician.

Besides the frustration and the time wasted it meant that his treatment was ultimately postponed for nearly five months. The good news was that he chose an outstanding specialist who treated him with a specialized type of radiation therapy and now, two years later, he remains completely free of any symptoms and had no side effects. A good ending, but not a good beginning. It did not need to be that way and it will not be in the future when medical information is digitized and is readily transportable via the Internet to whomever needs to get it.

MEGATRENDS SURROUNDING DIGITIZED MEDICAL INFORMATION

Medical data will become digitized. It will occur in fits and starts during the next five to fifteen years because the incentives are not well aligned and we lack a basic infrastructure and vocabulary that everyone follows. But the trend is inevitable. Digitization will allow access to medical information at any time, at any place, and in so doing will greatly improve the quality and safety of medical care—your medical care. Digitization will assist continuity of care by providing the right information at the right time to allow for the correct choices in care. Telemedicine and distance medicine will prevail.

Digitization will allow for a shift in where care is delivered—more at the community hospital instead of the academic medical center; more by a nurse practitioner rather than by a physician; and more at home rather than in a doctor's office. You will have your medical information on a card in your wallet or available securely on the Internet or both. You will be able to automatically have critical medical data, such as blood sugar, sent to your provider, and your provider will be able to send you health alerts.

Data mining, possible once the information is digitized, becomes easy, inexpensive, and extremely valuable. Digitized information will mean that preventive medicine comes into its own because you can learn what you need to know and your doctor can be reminded or remind you of the need for a vaccine or a colonoscopy. With digitized information, the computer can be put to real work for you, the patient. The computer can organize data, mine

THE MEGATRENDS

■ Medical Data Will Become Digitized
— Access Anytime, Anyplace
— Improve Quality and Safety of Care
— Distance Medicine Becomes Common
— Personal Access to Your Data
— Simulation to Improve Clinical Judgement
— Data Mining Improves Public's Health

data, manipulate data, and help to manage the vast amounts of medical data. All of this will be to your medical advantage. And you will not need to be your own Federal Express or UPS service, collecting and transporting your information from specialist to specialist.

WHAT YOU SHOULD KNOW

I hope you will take away not only an understanding of how medical records will become digitized for your own personal benefit and that of your family, but at the same time gain an understanding of the hurdles that need to be overcome in the next few years as medical information enters the digital age.

The critical issues confronting the digitization of medical information are not technical so much as they are human. It is a different way of working—and medicine is rather traditional and slow to convert. The financial incentives to encourage physicians to want and demand electronic medical records are generally lacking, since most often physicians find that their productivity is reduced, not enhanced, at least at first. Different systems do not interact or interconnect with each other, some systems present too much information, others present too little information, and few present just what the individual health care provider really needs at that point in time.

But the benefits of the digitization of medical information are clear. Electronic prescribing will speed up the process, reduce errors, eliminate handwriting mistakes, and in the process, alert physicians to problems such as allergies and drug-drug interactions, while teaching as they assist. Digitized medical information will ultimately have a dramatic effect on health care and will transform medicine with records available anywhere, anytime, and instantly. Search algorithms similar to the type that Google and Yahoo use today will assist health care providers in finding the right information quickly from the mountain of collected information. Other technologies will bring the right information together at the right time in locations such as the operating room or the intensive care unit.

The medical record will become *your* record—your personal health record. This is a change of mind-set, but it is coming. We will each either carry a wallet-sized card with an embedded chip with our medical information, or some type of flash memory such as the military's new dog tags called the Personal Information Carrier. Or we will be able to access our information through the Internet, reaching out to any site where our records have been kept and pulling it all together no matter where we may be at the time.

With access come security issues, and these will have to be clearly addressed. But just as the banks have done with the ATM system, there's no question that it can be done with our health care information. Our health care providers will be able to reach us with alerts and updates. Through telemedicine consults can be done anyplace, anytime by an expert unencumbered by time and distance. Intensive care units can be monitored from a distance, as can our home monitors for blood sugar, blood pressure, or weight.

Telemedicine will allow for not only consultations among physicians and other health care providers, but also between health care provider and patient, such as with the Mr. Rounder concept. Indeed we will soon be in the era of the "digital" hospital. With this conversion of information to a digitized format, the opportunity for data mining and data analysis becomes more and more possible in a relatively easy, inexpensive fashion.

WHAT YOU CAN DO

During the next five to fifteen years, these advances will occur. In the meantime, remember that your medical information is just that, it is yours. So when you see a physician, ask for a copy of the record. If you have an imaging study done, such as a CAT scan, ask for a copy. No, do not ask for a copy of the films; just ask them to burn you a CD with the digitized information on it. Then you will have it if you need to ever show it to another specialist. Do the same with laboratory information, or at least get a copy of the report. Some health care practitioners will be resistant, but remember the basic concept: it is *your* health information, and in the end, *you* are paying for it. This is a shift in thinking in medicine, but it is a shift that really needs to occur.

In the meantime, also watch for technologies where you can get your medical information summarized into a digital format. The iHealthrecord (www.ihealthrecord.org), affiliated with the American Medical Association, may be one way to go. It is an Internet-based personal health record that includes security, encryption of data, and a record of anyone who views the data with their name, date, and time. You can record emergency contacts and medical information, such as medications, allergies, and medical conditions.

You set up a password for access, and only you can give out the password to a physician or hospital in order to use it. So this is a system where you enter the data and let others access it at your choosing. Hopefully, it will not be too long before the data will be there automatically for you, and you will not have to run around collecting your personal data for a group of different specialists, as did Susan Gerard. It will either be with you or accessible via the Internet for easy access. Then your job, like Susan's, would be what it is meant to be—to deal with the diagnosis neither of them wanted to have and begin to understand how they were going to be treated—not worry about transporting medical information.

There are many reasons why health care costs are rising rapidly. Among them are a broken insurance system in the US, a poorly functioning malpractice system, an aging population, inadequate numbers of primary care physicians in needed locations, overuse of the ER as a substitute for primary care, overuse of expensive technologies and drugs, an unwillingness to accept that death is inevitable, a dysfunctional public health system with lack of adequate preventative care, and a citizenry that all too often fails to employ adequate perusal of self care—diet, exercise, stress reduction, use of seat belts, no tobacco, alcohol in moderation, dental hygiene, needed vaccinations, and routine evaluations and screenings.

CHAPTER 8

The High Cost of Medicine—How Much Is Due to Our Megatrends?

There are many reasons why health care costs are rising rapidly. Among them are a broken insurance system in the USA, a poorly functioning malpractice system, an aging population, an inadequate number of primary care physicians in needed locations, overuse of the ER as a substitute for primary care, overuse of expensive technologies and drugs, an unwillingness to accept that death is imminent, a dysfunctional public health system, an overall lack of preventative care, and a citizenry that all too often fails to employ adequate personal care—diet, exercise, stress reduction, use of seat belts, no tobacco, alcohol only in moderation, dental hygiene, needed vaccinations, and routine evaluations and screenings.

That said, there is general agreement that new technologies, such as the ones discussed in this book, are major drivers of the increasing costs of health care, which have risen about 10 percent per year for many years and now represent about 15 percent or more of our gross domestic product. Further, it has been argued that technological advances in general always increase expenditures even if the cost per unit goes down. Cell phones are an example. The price of cell phones has gone down substantially over the past few years, but the total expenditures for cell phones and service have increased dramatically.

Laparoscopic surgery has reduced the costs of removing a gallbladder, but there are indications that more people are now having the surgery done, so that the total expenditures are up even as the individual cost has dropped. When my mother had a heart attack in the 1950s, she was put on bed rest for two weeks in the hospital and then sent home. During my first years in practice, a patient would be admitted to the much more expensive cardiac care unit after a heart attack. Its value was in catching *heart arrhythmias* (irregular heart rhythms) before they became fatal, with a much improved survival rate.

And today, a patient is taken immediately for angioplasty and stent placement and possibly cardiac bypass surgery. Survival is up, and equally importantly, the heart muscle is spared so there is better quality of life after discharge. But it is expensive—very expensive—without question.[1]

A reasonable question to ask is: Does all this new technology, much of which is exceptionally expensive, just increase the burden of health care costs or does it actually make a positive difference? Let's consider a few scenarios, using examples from our discussions earlier of genomics, devices, imaging, and interventional radiology.

For Lisa Worthington, who came to the emergency room with atypical chest pain, the fast CT scanner proved to be particularly valuable. First of all, it told her and her physician that she was not having a heart attack or other life-threatening disease. She and her family were reassured, and quickly. It meant that she could go home and return to her physician at her leisure for the appropriate diagnostic studies to detect her esophageal reflux. It also freed the ER staff from hours of observation and further testing.

What about screening for heart disease? The current method in relatively young and otherwise healthy people who develop chest pain with exercise is to do an electrocardiogram and stress test. Then if it is still unclear whether a coronary artery is obstructed, the patient may be sent for catheterization and an angiogram. But now with the CT scan, it is possible to see the coronary arteries quickly and noninvasively. I suspect that this will become the standard approach soon, but it does require a fast CT scanner.

Recall that the sixty-four-slice scanner is capable of submillimeter imaging, and the coronary arteries are about 5 mm wide. This may allow early diagnosis of coronary artery disease and hence the need to consider angioplasty and stenting before symptoms appear and require an emergent procedure. So the scan is expensive, but it allows for a quick and safe method to learn if the coronary arteries are diseased. But like cell phones and laparoscopic surgery, will it lead to even more therapeutic procedures?

Then there is screening for *pulmonary embolism*—a blood clot in the lungs, usually starting in the legs or lower abdomen and migrating along the veins to the lungs. The standard approach has been a ventilation/perfusion scan in nuclear medicine. This is a relatively slow procedure, and it tends to give ambiguous results. Alternatively, one can do a pulmonary angiogram, which means placing a catheter in one of the large veins and running it up to the heart, injecting contrast material, and then taking fluoroscopic movies. This is the gold standard for detecting emboli, but it is a somewhat invasive procedure, takes a fair amount of time, and is very expensive. But with the new CT scanners, it is possible within just a few a seconds to see if there is a blood clot in the pulmonary arteries. If the CT scan is negative, it basically rules out pulmonary embolus; and if it is positive, one can immediately begin appropriate treatment and skip either the ventilation/perfusion scan or the pulmonary angiogram.

From a cost perspective, it makes sense to do the most appropriate imaging immediately, regardless of expense, rather than proceed with the least expensive test first, hoping that it will give the needed answer. Just as computer software can assist in drug selection, a computer program will soon help select the best diagnostic test to get to the answer quickly and most inexpensively. In this way, you have the test you really need, the answer comes quickly, and treatment can proceed expeditiously.

But not everybody needs every expensive test. The sixty-four-slice CT scanner can produce marvelous images, but it is needed only for certain tests, such as looking at the coronary arteries. It is not needed for routine scans and indeed gives too much radiation to use without proper justification. Here is where physician judgment and the use of computerized algorithms will be critical to assure that the right test is used for the right reason at the right time.

Recall our discussion of the cardiac assist device implanted in Mr. Caspian's heart to tide him over until his heart could stabilize—if it could. It turned out that his heart could not get back to anywhere near adequate function, but the device was able to carry him for three months until a heart was available for transplant. He did well with the transplant and ultimately went back to work. No question his life was saved. The device he received was still experimental, so there was no charge for the procedure, but his overall cost of care, including the transplant, was many hundreds of thousands of dollars.

Given that he is doing well, individuals have to make their own judgments as to ultimate value. At some point the cost is just too much—period. If he had to pay out of pocket, I suspect his family would have agreed that it was worth it. But, of course, he did well, and that was not certain until after the fact. Others die during the procedure, shortly after, or never have a heart transplant become available. So it becomes a difficult judgment call each time.

And what about drugs? New pharmaceuticals have had a major impact on health and life, but many of the newer dugs are prohibitively expensive. The newest cancer drugs, especially those that are targeted therapies are very expensive, often hundreds of thousands of dollars per year. And in this case, the average length of time of survival is still rather short for diseases like lung and colon cancer. On the other hand, Gleevec has had a very major impact on survival and quality of life for those with chronic myelocytic leukemia.

Why are new drugs so expensive? Part of the reason is that it costs about $800 million to $1 billion to bring forth a new drug. This includes all of the research and development expenses to study it and then get it approved by the FDA or similar regulatory bodies in other countries. So the company either needs to have a large market or charge a high price per pill/shot/dose to cover these costs.

Other countries such as Canada, establish price controls. The company can sell at that price or not. Usually, they do so provided the price is somewhat above their marginal costs. But in America, we pay the full price set by the company. In effect, we pay for the developmental costs.

Sometimes a drug is grossly overused. Viagra and Nexium are examples that come to mind. Watching the commercials on the evening news during the past few years, I would assume that most viewers must have erectile dysfunction or esophageal acid reflux disease. Far more Viagra is sold to people who do not really need it than to those who have a medical condition like diabetes or prostate surgery that causes impotence. But despite high sales volume, the pharmaceutical firm maintains a high price—about ten dollars per pill last time I checked—because the drug is still on patent and because sales are brisk, despite the price and even despite competition from its newer cousins, which have an equally high price.

What about chronic esophageal acid reflux? Some of us do of course have this problem, but the idea of the ad is to get anyone with a few symptoms to ask his physician to prescribe the newest, best drug. But like erectile dysfunction, much acid reflux is caused by stress. The first step should be to correct the stress in both cases and, for reflux esophagitis, correct one's eating habits or to use simple methods such as reducing alcohol consumption, waiting a few hours after dinner before going to bed, and/or putting the head of your bed on blocks to help the acid stay downhill. But all too many prefer to go to the doctor and ask for the pill that will fix the problem, rather than address the fundamental issues. And that is just what the pharmaceutical company hopes for with its advertising. No mention is made, of course, that a similar drug for acid reflux exists that is over-the-counter, but much cheaper and just as effective.

A lot of the total cost of health care is expended for relatively few patients with advanced diseases that usually occur near the end of life. This fact is often used to say that the expenses are not worthwhile because the patient dies anyway. Or at least, someone should pay attention to excessive expenditures if there is no hope for cure. It is often a fair statement in that physicians and patients both tend to often want to try "one last shot" to see if it works.

A recent study from Harvard and the University of Michigan looked at the value of medical spending as it has increased over the last forty years.[2] Adjusted for inflation, the average expense per person for medical care was seven hundred dollars in 1960; and in 2000, it was six thousand dollars. That is a very big increase. So they tried to determine if the increase was worth it in terms of increased survival. In short, they compared the levels of costs in 1960 to today and compared that to the number of additional years of life lived, using some assumptions for how much of that increase was probably due to medical care.

One of their examples is that newborn life expectancy increased by nearly seven years during this forty-year period. In other words, a child born in 2000 will, on average, live seven years longer than a child born in 1960. Most of that was due to a reduction in cardiovascular deaths and a reduced rate of death during infancy, especially for those born prematurely. It turned out the lifetime incremental costs increased about $20,000 for each year of life gained. Most economists, policy makers, and probably you, would consider that a reasonable cost to incur.

At older ages, their study showed that it cost more to achieve each added year of life. So, for example, at age sixty-five, each added year of life cost about $85,000, still probably an acceptable cost. However, the rate of rise in that cost was great, meaning that today it costs about $145,000 to gain a year of life, whereas, from 1960 to 1970, an incremental year of life cost about $75,000.

Overall, medical spending has risen about 10 percent per year for many years now. The study's authors referred to other work, suggesting that this is primarily due to new approaches such as this book discusses. Why does it cost more to increase life span for the older individual? Probably because at some point, we all get ill with some form of chronic disease such as heart disease, cancer, diabetes, or stroke, and these chronic diseases have proven expensive to treat. But it is also important to consider that the measure should not be just added years of life, but improved quality of life.

Perhaps a patient with cancer lives only a few more months but during that time has less pain, less suffering, and generally enjoys the time with his or her family. Mr. Caspian is an example of someone with severe heart disease who is enjoying an excellent quality of life after his heart transplant that was made possible because a device kept him alive long enough for a heart to become available. And Mrs. Perkins had an expensive procedure done to cure her brain aneurysm, but she is essentially fine today with little residual effect, except a minor speech impediment that most cannot detect.

Many believe that there needs to be cost containment in medicine. Clearly there needs to be a system that encourages the use of those technologies, procedures, and drugs that can have a worthwhile benefit and that limits or discourages the use of those that are of little value. Here is an example of overuse of transplants. About fifteen years ago, there was a lot of interest in using intensive chemotherapy along with a bone marrow transplant to treat patients with advanced breast cancer. There were studies in progress, but the results were not yet available. Many women had heard about this approach and along with their physicians wanted to give it a try rather than die. So they petitioned their insurance companies to cover the procedure, often $100,000 or more, and essentially demanded access to the procedure.

Often these attempts reached the newspapers with sad stories of how cruel the insurance companies were to not approve payment. Then a few years later, the studies were completed, and it turned out that there was no added benefit from the transplant. Indeed, it not only cost a lot more money, but it also had many serious complications. Today, it is a procedure that is rarely used for women with breast cancer. The point, of course, is that all of us need to be willing to wait until the definitive studies are completed and demonstrate that a procedure, technology, or drug is or is not of added value. If it is, then it should be considered for use. But if it is not, then it should not be considered.

So I would concur with the authors of the study referred to above: on average, medical spending has risen a lot, but the return has risen as well. The big question is whether the return is worth the cost. The key, it seems to me, is for each physician to make reasonable judgments in concert with his or her patients and their families about the best approach to each disease problem. That can be as momentous as deciding on something like a transplant or a very expensive device/procedure; or as apparently mundane as deciding if an expensive drug is really better than the generic one or the older drug that is available over-the-counter—or if a drug is needed at all.

To return to the Viagra and Nexium examples, both are treatments for problems that often are related to chronic stress. Instead of trying to solve it with a pill, wouldn't it be better to try to address the root cause and modify the stresses that are leading to these syndromes? It would lead to better overall health today and tomorrow, improvement in the current problem, and it would be less expensive. But sometimes that is hard for us to do—"Just give me a pill, doc." I will discuss this more in the last chapter.

PART III

From the Past, Coming Full Circle

Part III addresses the astonishing resurgence of complementary and alternative medicine as a major element of overall medical care during the past few decades and suggests that these modalities increasingly will become a legitimate and important part of everyday health maintenance and disease modification.

CHAPTER 9

Complementary Medicine—Ancient Traditions Affecting the Future

I was walking down the halls of the University of Maryland Medical Center one day on my way to a meeting, when I passed one of our staff. I said the ritual, "How are you doing?" And he gave me the wrong answer. I was late for a meeting and really only expected to hear the usual, "Everything is fine." But not today.

"Terrible, just terrible." The look in his eyes told me I had to stop and inquire further. He had been having migraine headaches for a number of years, had seen multiple physicians, and was taking a variety of medications. But the migraines recently had become both more frequent and more severe and nothing seemed to help. He had gone to a good neurologist who had nothing more to recommend, so I offered a suggestion.

"Why don't you try complementary medicine? Let me send you to Dr. Brian Berman." Dr. Berman, a physician trained in family medicine, became dissatisfied some twenty years ago with his inability to alleviate a variety of chronic pain problems troubling his patients. He began to learn acupuncture and found it helped. He moved to London, where he continued his training in acupuncture and other traditional medicine techniques.

In the early 1990s, he returned to Baltimore with a matching grant of one million dollars from the Maurice Laing Foundation to establish a medical school-based program in complementary medicine, which would conduct research—both basic and clinical—into various complementary medicine approaches. I had been involved in helping him set up the program and had heard some positive patient comments before my encounter in the hallway with our staff member. So I called Dr. Berman and arranged for a visit.

A few weeks later, he stopped by my office to say that his life was fundamentally changed. "It's like a new lease on life. I am actually living again!

Dr. Berman used acupuncture, which had a fairly immediate effect, and then he taught me relaxation techniques that I have been using regularly, and it helps a lot." Comments like these are not uncommon from individuals with various types of chronic pain problems after they are treated with complementary medicine.

How does complementary medicine, which employees techniques many millennia old, fit into a book on the future of medicine? Their use is indeed developing into a major trend in this country and many others. People are voting with their feet and their pocketbooks. They visit complementary medicine practitioners in ever-increasing numbers, and they pay for most of it with cash, since it is usually not reimbursed by health insurance. It is a significant megatrend in medical care. Increasingly, we are learning how these treatments work or if they work at all. Research dollars are available to learn what works and what does not, and even more important, why something works when it does.

In 1993 Dr. Eisenberg and his colleagues at Harvard Medical School published an article in the *New England Journal of Medicine* on a survey completed in 1990.[1] They found that 33 percent of those surveyed had used one or more complementary medicine therapies during the previous year. Seventy percent of these individuals did not tell their physicians about this use.

In general, patients sought complementary therapies for chronic conditions, such as pain or arthritis. The authors then generalized their findings to the entire American population. This would suggest that there were more visits to complementary medicine practitioners (425 million) than to primary care physicians (338 million) in 1990. They estimated the total cost in the United States to be $13.9 billion. Of this, only about $3.6 billion would have been covered by insurance with the remainder, about $10.3 billion, spent out of pocket.

TERMINOLOGY AND THE USE OF COMPLEMENTARY MEDICINE

The terminology is confusing. Many use the term *alternative medicine,* which to me implies the avoidance of conventional medicine and practitioners. Complementary medicine, on the other hand, implies working in conjunction with conventional medicine and practitioners. Some use the term *integrative* medicine to suggest the integration of both complementary and "Western" medicine. Whatever term is used—alternative, integrative, or complementary—the science has been observational, rather than experimental, in the past.

Until recently, medical schools did not teach these techniques, and physicians trained in Western medicine generally have not accepted complementary practitioners. Many complementary medicine techniques exist, but until recently, these techniques were not accepted since they lacked a scientific basis. In the last decade, however, high-quality research is beginning to evaluate them.

Stand in the checkout line at your local supermarket, and the covers of many magazines feature various alternative or complementary medicine techniques. And if you go to the local bookstore, a large section is devoted to alternative medicine. In 1997, the *Wall Street Journal* estimated that chiropractic, acupressure, reflexology, and other similar services represented a $98 billion market in the United States, up 69 percent in less than ten years. Meanwhile, multiple medical schools and medical centers began to develop curricula and programs in complementary medicine. Among the early adaptors were Harvard Medical School and Beth Israel Hospital in Boston, Massachusetts; Stanford Medical School in Palo Alto, California; and the University of Maryland Medical School in Baltimore, Maryland.

Insurance commonly covers chiropractic and occasionally covers acupressure. But it rarely covers massage, support groups, or herbal remedies. Some innovative insurers are seeing value, such as AETNA, which will reimburse for the Ornish Cardiac Program that I will describe later. But, by and large, third-party payers have been reluctant to commit to complementary medicine techniques.

Complementary medicine is commonly practiced and not viewed negatively by physicians in the United Kingdom and other European countries, such as Finland, the Netherlands, Germany, and France. About a decade ago, Japan estimated that the Japanese spend about $1.3 billion per year for *kampo* (herbal) remedies. But in Japan, Western medicine has staked out a strong position, and at least until recently, the kampo and the Western medicine practitioners rarely interacted. In China, of course, traditional Chinese medicine is common and indeed practiced more than what we call Western medicine. In India, the dominant medical approach is what is called *Ayurveda*, which is an alternative method as well.

SCIENTIFIC STUDIES OF COMPLEMENTARY MEDICINE

The National Institutes of Health created the National Center for Complementary and Alternative Medicine (NCCAM) under the leadership of a highly respected infectious disease investigator, Stephen E. Strauss, MD, to study alternative and complementary medicine in a scientific manner. (See the NCCAM web site at www.nccam.nih.gov.) The Center offers grants to institutions to study diseases, such as cancer and musculoskeletal pain, to see how complementary medicine might be of benefit.

The Center is heavily engaged in multiple studies to assess the scientific validity of complementary medicine practices. Some studies have shown positive results (acupuncture for osteoarthritis pain) and some have been negative (St. John's wort for depression). The point is to learn what does and what does not work, in a manner that is scientific and unbiased.

COMPLEMENTARY MEDICINE PRACTICES

Complementary medicine practices include acupuncture, herbal medicine, support groups, and a variety of mind-body approaches, such as meditation, the relaxation response, creative visualization, and prayer, as well as touch therapies, such as massage.

Acupuncture

Acupuncture goes back to ancient China, where fish bones were used as needles and over hundreds of years practitioners discovered certain sites that had a beneficial effect for different problems. Scientific studies prove acupuncture is valuable for a variety of musculoskeletal pain syndromes, such as those caused by osteoarthritis.

One study treated individuals with osteoarthritis of the knee with the best available therapy and then randomized them to receive either real or sham acupuncture. Those who received the real acupuncture used fewer pain medications and had greater knee mobility than did those who received the sham acupuncture.[2] Similarly a study of pain following wisdom tooth extraction showed that those who received acupuncture reported less pain and used fewer medications postoperatively. As I mentioned, migraine responds to acupuncture as well, and acupuncture and acupressure are quite effective at stress reduction.

Postoperative nausea and vomiting can be reduced by the use of acupuncture, as can the nausea and vomiting caused by cancer chemotherapy.

Acupuncture also is valued as part of the treatment for stress management. A friend called early one morning to say that she had severe pain in her neck that radiated into her shoulder and was truly incapacitating. Based on the description, I called an orthopedist who agreed to show up at his office thirty minutes early, so that he could fit her in. She was unable to lift her arm up directly perpendicular to her body. With that observation and the rest of the examination along with an X-ray, he diagnosed a bone spur in her neck. It was pressing on a nerve, causing the pain and also blocking the nerve impulses to her arm so that she could not raise it.

Long story short is that she was hospitalized, put in traction, and given some muscle relaxants. The pain subsided and function returned to her arm. Two neurosurgeons examined her and determined that she did not need surgery, but told her to continue physical therapy, take pain medicines, and use muscle relaxants as necessary. Although this worked, the symptoms never totally abated, and she spent weekends "catching up." It was really affecting the quality of her life.

I wondered if Dr. Berman might be able to help her, so I called and asked if he had ever dealt with patients like this. "Oh, yes, quite a few times, and I usually get pretty good results" was the answer. So she went to see him, and as with the other patient I described, he used acupuncture and also taught her the relaxation response of Dr. Herbert Benson. (See the Mind-Body Techniques section that follows.) She told me that as she traveled home that first day, she commented to her husband, "I'm not certain exactly what just happened, but I know that something has fundamentally changed in my body."

She received acupuncture three days the first week, two days a week for the next two weeks, and then once a week thereafter for a few weeks. After four weeks, her symptoms were entirely gone, and she was off all medication—the first time in more than a year. In the ensuing twelve years, she has had occasional flare-ups of symptoms, which she resolved herself with stretching and the relaxation response, although on one occasion she went back to Dr. Berman for a "tune-up." Such is the power of complementary medicine in certain settings.

Acupuncture

- Osteoarthritis
- Low Back Pain
- Postoperative Nausea/ Discomfort
- Pain after Wisdom Tooth Extraction
- Migraine
- Stress
- Chronic Pain Syndromes

How does acupuncture work? No one knows for sure, but the research to date suggests that it affects the regulatory functions of the nervous system. One of these functions regulates the production of painkilling biochemicals such as endorphins. Another theory is that acupuncture may adjust the balance between our sympathetic and parasympathetic nervous systems, and it may also affect our immune system. Brain chemistry appears to be affected as well, with the release of compounds called *neurotransmitters* and *neurohormones*, which in turn affect those parts of our nervous system related to sensation and involuntary body functions, such as blood pressure and body temperature. It apparently also has some powerful nonspecific effects as well as its specific effects, as shown in a study of chronic neck pain.[3]

Touch Therapies and Massage

The form of touch therapy that most of us are familiar with, or at least have heard of, is massage.

The word comes from Arabic meaning "to stroke," and ancient records show massage use more than three thousand years ago in China and forty-two hundred years ago in Egypt. Hippocrates was a strong advocate during his time. But it fell into disrepute in the West, beginning in the Middle Ages when the Catholic Church denounced massage as "the work of the devil." By the mid-twentieth century, massage was often associated with prostitution. Massage took on a negative aura that began to change only recently.

Good evidence documents that massage can be quite helpful with premature infants. In comparing neonates treated with massage versus those not treated, the massaged infants became more alert, more active, and more responsive.

Touch Therapies—Massage

- Premature Infants – Home Sooner
- Asthma – Less Medication
- Anxiety – Reduction
- Stress – Reduction
- Muscular Aches and Discomfort – Relief
- Migraine Headache – Relief

They gained weight nearly 50 percent faster than the nonmassaged infants, they slept more deeply, and they left the neonatal intensive care unit six days sooner with about a $10,000 lower hospital bill. Some evidence shows that asthma can be improved with massage, and that immune function can be improved to some degree in those with HIV infection. Burn victims have lessened anxiety with massage, and massage can help individuals with depression. Massage is useful for migraine headaches and is particularly useful for reducing stress. There is even a recent report that massage during the last weeks of pregnancy can reduce the need for episiotomies during delivery.[4] Of course, massage is useful for relieving the aches and discomfort of exercise, whether from hiking, biking, or working out in the gym.

Herbal Medicine

Many of us are inherently suspicious of herbal medicine, but the truth is, until recently, most of our medications came from plants. A good example is digitalis, the drug used for control of certain heart irregularities and for heart failure. Digitalis comes from the foxglove plant and was found by William Withering in England in 1785 to have value for heart patients. In the mid-twentieth century the pharmaceutical companies discovered the active ingredient and chemically synthesized it.

Herbal Medicine

- Does the Compound Work?
- Does it Lack Impurities?
- Is the Dose Consistent?

This had the advantage of ensuring that the compound was pure and that each tablet had exactly the same amount of drug in it. Herein are the three key issues with herbal medicines: Do they really work? (Withering did studies with patients to suggest a real effect.) Does the herbal prescription have other compounds in it that may cause problems—is it pure? (A chemically synthesized drug is guaranteed pure.) Does the remedy given to you have the same dose as the last time? Often it does not. (The chemically synthesized drug has a guaranteed dose.)

The problem with herbal extracts is that one can never be sure of the purity or of the dose.[5] My sassafras tea that I steeped for a few minutes may work great, but if you use a different root and steeped it differently, it may not work. The other issue is whether the plant or herb contains other co-active or inactive compounds that may have other effects, both good and bad. Western medicine, with its preference for pharmaceutically manufactured chemical compounds as drugs, has the benefit of purity, known dosage, and extensive clinical testing for effectiveness and safety. And it is all reviewed and approved by the Food and Drug Administration. Over-the-counter herbal remedies are regulated for safety (to a somewhat lesser standard than drugs), but not for effectiveness.

If you have ever seen a field of the beautiful light yellow flowers of St. John's wort, you would intuitively feel that it must be a good treatment for depression. Although used extensively, recent well-controlled studies suggest that St. John's wort is, in fact, of little use for major depression, although there might be some efficacy for mild, transient depression. Similarly, studies of *Echinacea* for the common cold have not shown any degree of efficacy, but many people swear by it. These and others continue to be used, such as garlic for hypertension, ginseng as a general tonic, and dong quai for menopausal symptoms, probably because it contains some estrogenlike properties. *Ginkgo biloba* is said by some to improve mental acuity, slow the onset of Alzheimer's, and generally augment memory, but none of this has ever been proven. The NCCAM is conducting large-scale controlled trials to address the potential uses of ginkgo; these will be completed in a few years. Meanwhile, a recent study supported by NCCAM has shown benefit for selected patients with moderate to severe pain of osteoarthritis when treated with glucosamine/chondroitin sulfate. This compound has been used for years by many but until now its value was never clarified. And even here, it was not useful for all patients, just a subset. These trials and others are discussed on the NCCAM Web site noted previously.

Mind-Body Techniques

The journalist Bill Moyers developed a television series followed by a book entitled *Healing and the Mind*.[6] It is a good book to read to better understand how the mind and body work together for health and for disease. I will review a few of the mind-body techniques that alternative and complementary medicine practitioners use, including meditation, the relaxation response, visualization, guided imagery, support groups, and prayer. Let's start with meditation.

Meditation. Although seemingly rather mysterious, meditation is rather simple in concept although difficult in practice. The idea is to focus our attention and dispel the thoughts that are normally in our minds. Meditation can result in a state of pleasant relaxation with mental calmness.[7]

Studies of meditators have shown major changes in brain activity. Functional MRI and PET scans have both shown that those who meditate regularly have significant differences in the way their brain functions during meditation. For example, the Dalai Lama arranged for eight highly experienced and trained meditators to be studied at the Keck Laboratory for Functional Imaging and Behavior at the University of Wisconsin. Ten student volunteers with a week's training served as controls. All were told to meditate on "unconditional loving-kindness and compassion."

The brains of the highly experienced meditators responded much differently than did those of the students. The Tibetan monks induced sustained, high levels of gamma waves in their brains. In fact, there was a "dose response" with the most experienced practitioners having the most change in brain wave activity, as measured with extensive electroencephalographic testing. They were also tested with functional MRI (see the chapter on imaging). This showed that the major changes were in the prefrontal cortex, which is the area of the brain just above and behind the forehead. Earlier work had shown that this area is associated with a sense of positivity and happiness. Other earlier work had indicated that this type of brain wave change correlates with focus, memory, and consciousness. The lead scientist, Richard Davidson, concluded that meditation changes the way the brain works, with more change with more experience. This suggests that we can alter how our brain functions and control that function for the benefit of our health.[8]

Studies suggest that meditation may, via our brains, adjust our autonomic nervous system. This is the two-part system of the sympathetic and parasympathetic nervous systems. The former prepares us for action such as when we walk across the street and see a car rushing at us. Our heart beats faster and stronger, breathing increases, and muscles are ready to run. The latter system allows our body to rest with a decreased heart rate and blood pressure, relaxed muscle tone, and slowed breathing. Meditation is believed to augment the parasympathetic system and tone down the sympathetic system thus leading to a relaxed, comfortable state.

There is an ancient Chinese system of martial arts called Tai Chi Chih. It inspired a series of twenty gentle, soft, slow movements that most of us can perform, even the elderly. Many do this as a wellness exercise at local athletic clubs or neighborhood centers. There is a study showing that regular Tai Chi actually boosts your immunity to the virus that causes herpes zoster (shingles). Since as many as 20 percent of normal people over the age of sixty develop this painful and often disfiguring infection, any technique to reduce the possibility is welcome.[9] Besides, it is fun and those that do it report much improved mobility and pleasant relaxation. But don't forget the new vaccine for shingles discussed in the vaccine chapter.

The Relaxation Response. In the mid-1970s, a cardiologist at Harvard, Herbert Benson, MD, was studying the treatment of hypertension. One day some Tibetan monks came to his office and said that they could help him reduce high blood pressure rather simply with meditation. He was skeptical but did some work with them, and he was satisfied that meditation would reduce blood pressure and have a general calming influence. He wanted a simplified meditation technique that he could easily teach his patients. He developed something he called the *relaxation response,* which is in essence to sit quietly and close your eyes. Then breathe slowly and deeply with the diaphragm and silently say a word with each exhalation. Any word will do; it can be as simple as saying the word *one.* Throughout all of this, relax completely. And whenever your mind wanders, as it surely will, just bring it back to your breathing and saying your word. This has proven to be easy to do and has been effective in reducing blood pressure and in reducing blood pressure medication requirements.[10]

Visualization. Visualization and guided imagery are related mind-body techniques. With creative visualization, an individual seeks a quiet resting state in a semi-meditative mode in which they imagine themselves as healthy, free of disease, free of certain habits—such as smoking or overeating—or enthused about positive attributes such as exercise. The concept is that if one repetitively embeds a desired state into the subconscious mind, the mind-body connections will work toward that state in an ongoing fashion. Guided imagery is a similar technique in which the patient imagines elements of the body actively affecting a disease; for example, macrophages and natural killer cells are imagined as moving toward the tumor and destroying it.

Support Groups. Support groups have proven to be extremely helpful to patients with a variety of different illnesses. Studies show that a patient's major concern is that of dying alone, either literally or figuratively. The second major concern is having unmanaged pain. Multiple studies of support groups that have looked at quality of life have shown that the quality of life has been much improved by the use of simple support groups. Patients are better able to cope with pain, have less psychological distress, reduced anxiety, reduced depression, and increased physical activity. Support groups clearly have great value.

If you think about it, complementary medicine practitioners usually spend more time with their patients than do most physicians; they spend more time addressing symptoms and more time focusing on concerns. This is one reason so many people go to complementary medicine practitioners. Physicians who get their patients enrolled and engaged in support groups can add a lot to their relationship with their patient. Support groups start by teaching coping skills—coping, for example, with various medical team members. Then patients learn self-pain management, often aided by self-hypnosis as well as relaxation and problem-solving techniques to help deal with the problems of their illness. Having a good handle on these types of coping skills can make an individual much more comfortable with his illness and more at ease with his health care providers.

A rather famous study was done at Stanford Medical School by Dr. Spiegel, a medical oncologist who was taking care of patients with metastatic breast cancer.[11] He wanted to determine if support groups with psychosocial therapy would aid his patients' quality of life. He took eighty-six women and randomly allocated half of them to be part of a support group with psychosocial intervention. Those who were in the intervention group went to a weekly supportive group therapy session that lasted about ninety minutes. They were taught self-hypnosis for pain, along with coping skills, and had the opportunity to discuss their problems among themselves.

The patients in both groups continued with their standard oncologic care. This study was designed to address psychological distress and pain management and to look at quality of life. It was not designed to study survival. Over time, Dr. Spiegel was able to demonstrate that the patients who were part of the support group experienced decreased anxiety and decreased pain and, as a result, an improved overall quality of life. An interesting side observation was that patients in the support group survived, on average, quite a bit longer (thirty-seven months) than did those who were in the control group (nineteen months).

When this was published, unfortunately, most people focused on the survival data and began to argue whether the study was well designed to address survival issues. Dr. Spiegel himself said that was not the point of the study and that the real issue was quality of life—which was clearly improved. Since then, other studies have tried to look at the survival issue, but I would emphasize the importance of the support group to improve quality of life by decreasing anxiety and pain and improving the ability to cope and interact with health care providers.

A more recent study allocated patients with breast cancer to one of three groups: standard care, standard care with support sessions, or standard care with imagery sessions. Quality of life and immune function was then measured. Compared to those in the standard care group, those who had support sessions demonstrated better coping skills and a greater sense of meaning to life. Those in the imagery sessions were found to have less stress, more vigor, and more social and functional quality of life.[12]

Prayer. Many of you reading this book pray regularly and consider it a normal and important part of your life. You may not be aware that some interesting experiments have looked at the use of prayer and medicine. Some studies suggest that those who pray or consider themselves religious do better after surgery. But what if someone prays for you?—intercessory prayer or prayer at a distance. In 1988, Dr. R. C. Byrd published a paper on the use of prayer for patients who had had a heart attack.[13] He studied 383 patients who were admitted to the coronary care unit of San Francisco General Hospital with a *myocardial infarction* (heart attack). All patients received equivalent care, but half—based on their assigned hospital chart number—were prayed for and half were not.

This study met the strict scientific criteria of being prospective and randomized and double blind, the latter meaning that Dr. Byrd and his colleagues did not know which patients were being prayed for and which patients were not until after the study was completed and the results analyzed. A group of five to seven people prayed at home and had no personal knowledge of the patient. They had no specific instruction other than to pray once a day for the patients.

The results were striking. Fewer patients in the group receiving prayer developed pulmonary edema (six vs. eighteen). Fewer patients required being placed on a respirator (zero vs. twelve), and fewer required antibiotics (three vs. eighteen). These three factors were all statistically significant. Fewer patients died in the group that was prayed for, but this difference was not statistically significant, meaning that the differences could have been due to chance. So prayer seemed to benefit these individuals with heart attacks.

A follow-up study in Kansas City, Missouri, in 1998 found that intercessory prayer benefited heart attack patients as well. They studied 990 patients admitted to the coronary care unit. The patients did not know that they were being prayed for. At the end of 50 weeks, those who were prayed for showed positive improvement compared to the others.[14] L. Dossey, MD, is a physician who has written several books related to complementary medicine including the implications of spirituality on healing.[15] He notes that more than 100 clinical studies have concluded that intercessory prayer can benefit health. Although not all have been grounded in strong scientific method, many have.

As I write this chapter, a new study that looked at 1,802 patients having open-heart surgery has been published. Dr. Herbert Benson led the study.[16] There were three groups of patients: one group was not prayed for, one was prayed for but was not told so, and one group was prayed for and was told that they were being prayed for. Prayers were offered by two Catholic groups and by one Protestant group. Each prayed in his or her own manner but was encouraged to use the phrase "for a successful surgery, healthy recovery, and no complications."

There were no major differences in the first two groups, but the group that knew they were being prayed for had more, rather than fewer, complications. The investigators considered that perhaps the latter group felt under some level of stress that they "should" do better since they were told they were being prayed for. But I doubt that the results of this study will discourage you from praying for your loved ones nor from hoping that you will be prayed for if you need surgery or have a serious illness.

The Spindrift Foundation is an interesting nonprofit in Salem, Oregon.

They have been studying prayer in a scientific fashion for many years. One of the studies that I find fascinating shows that if you plant two groups of seeds and pray for just one group, it is that group that does better. Length of prayer seems to be important, and extended prayer led to twice as many seeds germinating. The experience of the person praying was important; those with more experience were able to get more of their seeds to germinate.

They also learned that nondirected prayer was twice as effective as directed prayer (the difference between praying "make my seeds grow" versus "thy will be done"). Prayer seems to work best when the person praying does so from a loving and kind perspective—truly caring for the seeds but accepting God's will.

We have lots to learn and in this very scientific and technologic era in which we live, we are learning that some of the basics handed down to us through the generations have a lot of validity.

PUTTING IT ALL TOGETHER

Let me try to put some of these various complementary medicine approaches together by describing a study done by Dr. Dean Ornish and his colleagues.[17] Dr. Ornish is a cardiologist trained at Harvard Medical School and Massachusetts General Hospital who now works in the San Francisco area. He became interested during medical school at Baylor in whether risk factor modification could have a major impact on his patients who had significant heart disease. Indeed, he wondered whether he could actually reverse some of the changes in the coronary arteries through risk factor modification. He took a group of patients and documented their coronary artery disease through the use of an arteriogram done in the cardiac catheterization laboratory. He also had access to PET scanners and did PET scans as well to look at heart wall muscle function. Having documented the degree of coronary artery disease, he then established a program that included stress management, diet, exercise, and group support.

The diet was vegetarian, low in fat and cholesterol. Patients received help in quitting smoking, and they did mild to moderate aerobic exercise three hours per week. I need to emphasize that the low-fat diet was indeed a very low-fat diet, but Dr. Ornish and his colleagues helped design tasty, easily prepared meals. To reduce stress each patient did Hatha yoga stretching and meditated an hour per day.

There were regular support group sessions. After five years, the angiograms and PET scans were repeated. The result was rather dramatic. The angiograms of many patients showed reductions in stenosis in the coronary arteries and the size and severity of the perfusion abnormalities on PET scanning decreased, meaning that their heart muscle function had improved.

Dr. Ornish and his colleagues were able to show that an aggressive program of reducing the known risk factors to coronary artery disease had a substantive measurable impact.

What does this mean to you? Well, if you are one of those who know you have high cholesterol, are overweight, your blood pressure is high, or you are heavily stressed and you are not certain if working on this would really have an impact, then here is proof that it does.

The problem is that we do not know which individual items within the Ornish program were most important. Do you have to do them all? Was it the very low-fat diet or was it the meditation? I guess the bottom line is that we may not know which elements are most important but they all make good sense, so if you already have coronary artery disease, entering a program like this is a sensible course. And by the way, it does need to be a *program,* because you need the assistance of trained advisors to help you with the diet, the meditation, the support group issues, and so forth.

RECAP

To recap what we have explored, complementary medicine is used commonly by individuals but usually without their physician's knowledge. Until recently most of the complementary medicine techniques had not been subjected to scientific evaluations although that is certainly changing now.

The clinical studies to date have shown that a variety of techniques are helpful in specific situations, such as acupuncture for the pain of osteoarthritis and massage for premature infants. Meanwhile, anecdotal evidence and thousand-year traditions suggest efficacy for many other techniques. That said, not everything that is purported to work does so, and you can end up spending a lot of money needlessly. But certainly acupuncture can be considered for both relaxation and pain management; herbal therapies can have a role including a good hot cup of tea for relaxation; meditation for stress reduction; support groups to improve quality of life; massage for muscle relaxation and a general sense of well-being; and, of course, prayer for spiritual needs.

A HOLISTIC MODEL FOR MEDICAL CARE

True holistic medical care needs to start with what we think of as standard or science-based medicine, the so-called Western tradition of medicine today. To that is added symptom-based therapy, such as the relief of pain; attention to preventive medicine, such as diet, exercise, stress reduction, and massage; and attention to psycho-social needs, which would include financial counseling and home health care when necessary, as well as attention to spiritual needs such as meditation and prayer. Physicians need not be expert in all aspects of this holistic approach to care, but they do need to be able to connect the patient and the patient's family with those who are.

In the chapter on genomics, I suggest there is a new developing paradigm for medicine, which will take us from today's "diagnose and treat" to tomorrow's "predict and prevent."

Another new paradigm for medicine is that we will bring the physician and the patient back together again in a meaningful fashion with a holistic approach to care made possible, in part, by the developing trends in technology that have been reviewed in this book.

The bigger reasons for this paradigm change will be that physicians and others will get a better sense of professionalism in their education and training[18] and that patients will demand holistic care—by frequenting those who practice it and avoiding others. Physicians learn quickly when it affects their pocketbooks, just like everyone else.

MEGATRENDS RELATED TO COMPLEMENTARY MEDICINE

Society is less and less satisfied with the brief encounters and lack of personal attention that we receive all too often in today's health care environment. Many feel that simpler care is better care. As a result, patients are voting with their feet and their pocketbooks and using complementary medical practitioners and approaches more and more often.

Concurrently, physicians, nurses, and other health care providers are learning more about these ancient practices and are putting them to work or, at least, referring their patients to trusted practitioners in the community. And at the same time there are now sound scientific studies ongoing to test and understand which techniques work, for what and how. During the next five to fifteen years, I believe we will see a flowering of complementary medicine practices, procedures, and practitioners and a true integration of Western scientific medicine with complementary medicine. With it will be a much more holistic approach to care where the patient—and not the disease—is the focus of attention. A much more "personal" form of personalized medicine which will in its way be a transformational megatrend.

THE MEGATRENDS

- Patients Attracted to Complementary Medicine (CM)
- Caregivers Learning About CM
- Complementary Medicine Will Flower
  Practioners
  Procedures
  Practices
- CM and Western/Scientific Medicine Will Become Much More Integrated
- A More Holistic Approach to Medicine Will Ensue

WHAT YOU SHOULD KNOW

You should be aware of the basic types of complementary medicine practices such as acupuncture, herbal medicines, massage, and meditation. You should also know at least something about what practices work for some common ailments—such as acupuncture for chronic and acute pain; meditation for high blood pressure; support groups for those with chronic, severe diseases; and massage for neonates. And you should know what you want from your health care practitioners—total care, holistic care, personal care. The best science and all the latest tests and treatments may be important (and they certainly are), but they are not sufficient—and you should not be satisfied with anything less.

WHAT YOU CAN DO

Do consider the use of complementary medicine techniques and practitioners. Be wary of physicians who disparage their use or efficacy, but at the same time do not expect complementary medicine to cure cancer or strokes. Rather look to these practices and practitioners to relieve suffering, improve outlook and functioning, and help you enjoy a better, more productive and fulfilled life. Complementary medicine is best when used in conjunction with your physician's overall plan for your care—not as an alternative to good medical care from a competent, knowledgeable, and compassionate physician.

Look to practitioners that your physician recommends, just as you would a specialist or a surgeon. Check out their credentials and their experience, just as you would a new internist or pediatrician. And finally, you deserve holistic medical care and nothing less. So find yourself a competent and caring physician who respects you as a whole person and not just as a patient with a series of symptoms. You will get better care and you will feel better about it in the process.

PART IV

It Is Up to You

Part IV addresses the critical issue of patient safety, what is being done to improve safety, what needs to be done now, and how you can push the system to effect the needed changes. Then follows a discussion of how you can maintain your own health and, as a result, benefit from the remarkable advances in medical care that this book has outlined.

CHAPTER 10

Preventable Medical Errors— A National Disgrace

We all assume that our health care provider will not make mistakes, at least not when treating us. But doctors, nurses, physical therapists, pharmacists, and the rest are all human and endowed with a common characteristic, namely, they all make mistakes just like the rest of humanity. Certainly, no one comes to work in the morning determined to make a mistake; indeed, a lot of effort and energy goes into not making a mistake—but it still happens. In this chapter, we will review why errors occur and what is being done to prevent them in the future.

All of us make mistakes. Sometimes it is just forgetfulness like not bringing home a quart of milk for dinner. "I forgot" doesn't satisfy your spouse, but indeed, it was just that simple. Consider when you were in school and had a major exam. You prepared hard and well, found the test not too difficult, checked all your answers carefully, and left the test site convinced you did great. But the score came back much lower than you expected, and you realize that you made a bunch of dumb mistakes. *How could that be?* you asked yourself. You were attentive, alert, determined, and focused, yet you still made enough mistakes to get a lower grade. This happened to me for the final exam in freshman math in college; I couldn't believe that I made such dumb mistakes. I really knew the material, but it didn't matter—I got a lower grade, and obviously I still remember it today.

What's needed is a system to catch errors before or just after they are made. That is why we check the addition of a column of numbers by adding up instead of down. Just adding down again may well replicate the mistake we made the first time, but when we add up, we see the problem differently. Think of this as a simple system. It is the sort of system that I ignored during my math test, to my dismay! Systems are needed in hospitals to prevent medical errors from occurring. They exist, but better systems can be more effective in preventing avoidable errors.

Imagine the following examples of mistakes—made by bright, dedicated individuals with their patient's best interest at heart—that should not have happened. But they did.

A tiny premature infant was in the neonatal intensive care unit with the best doctors and nurses, all well trained and experienced. The baby was on a ventilator, had an intravenous line in place, and was fed through a feeding tube. At about 5:00 in the morning the nurses routinely change all the various tubing; this is done to reduce the chance of infection. It is done at this time of day because there is less activity—the parents are home, the doctors are not present, and the phones are not ringing. At 6:30 one morning, the monitor indicated that this infant had a rising heart rate. The nurses could not find a reason but summoned the pediatricians who, likewise, could find no cause.

About an hour later, someone realized that the baby's feeding tube had been inadvertently switched for the intravenous tube; formula was going directly into the baby's veins. What had happened at 5:00 a.m. to allow this error to occur? The nurse on duty that night had twelve years of experience with premature infants, was highly respected, was a role model for new nurses, and had a perfect attendance record. The nurse had not been distracted—no other emergencies, no phone calls. The nurse was not overloaded with patients and was not covering for anyone else who might have left for a break, snack, or to run an errand. In essence, everything was fine at that time on that shift; no extraneous reasons caused the nurse to make this mistake. It was "just" a human error, albeit a serious one. Indeed, the baby died.

This episode was a wake-up call for me on patient safety. I was chief operating officer of the hospital system at the time and was about to become CEO of the flagship academic medical center. A new chair of the board of trustees had just taken over, and he asked to spend time after each board meeting, touring the hospital and learning more about patient care. On the first tour, we went to the neonatal intensive care unit where the head nurse took us from room to room. The first room had the "growers," medical slang for somewhat premature infants that needed some time in the hospital before going home. The baby that President and Mrs. John F. Kennedy lost forty years ago would have fit into this group, she explained. But nowadays, essentially all of these infants survive and live perfectly normal lives.

From there, we went to each of three rooms that held successively smaller infants. At the last room the babies could only be termed *tiny*—no larger than a man's hand. Indeed, it seemed amazing that they could live, even with all of the medical and nursing help available. The chairman, standing by an incubator and looking down at one of these infants, asked if this child could possibly survive.

"Yes," was the reply, "this baby has no congenital problems, so we will just need to keep up with using the respirator, giving it IV fluids, and feeding it through the feeding tube for a few months. Then it should be fine."

I could tell that the board chair was amazed, as was I, and that he really felt good. Here he was, volunteering a lot of his time, and now he could have the satisfaction that "his" hospital was doing great things for the citizenry.

Two days later, I was called about the premature infant that had had the tubes reversed. It was the same infant that we had talked about on the tour. I knew I had to call the chairman, but I dreaded doing so; it would be a real downer for him. And how could I explain that it was "just a mistake," terrible, but a mistake nonetheless? I had thought that we paid attention to safety, but upon reflection and some investigation, it became abundantly clear that giving real, intensive, and sustained attention to patient safety is critical for any hospital CEO. Of course, we all care about safety and our patients' welfare, but I can state from experience that most of us simply do not realize what needs to be done and done differently to make a real difference. I will address what these needs are shortly, but first let's consider some other preventable medical errors.

■ ■ ■

At one of the nation's preeminent cancer centers, Dana Farber Cancer Center in Boston, a medical oncology fellow (a fellow is someone who has graduated from medical school, finished a three-year internal medicine residency, is eligible and may have now taken the board certification examination, and has decided to take an additional three years of training in medical oncology, i.e., is well trained but not yet long on experience) orders a combination of drugs to treat a patient's metastatic (widespread) breast cancer. One of the drugs, cyclophosphamide, is requested at a high dose as per his understanding of an institutional research protocol in which the patient has agreed to participate. The pharmacist believes the dose is too high and must be miscalculated and so calls the physician. The physician recalculates it and calls back that his initial order is correct. The pharmacist is still concerned and, together with two other pharmacists, reviews the protocol. They conclude that the protocol dosing schedule is somewhat confusing, but that the physician is apparently correct.

The drug is prepared, but the nurse challenges the dose. The pharmacist explains the steps just taken, so the nurse administers it. The protocol calls for the drug to be repeated each day for three days; the patient receives the drug each day. Later, she develops heart failure and ultimately dies. Meanwhile, a second patient receives the same course of therapy and is left with severe heart failure. No one realizes the dose error yet, so the adverse events are not connected with an overdose. But the first patient was a reporter for the *Boston Globe*, and a colleague wrote a series of investigative stories that shook the cancer center to its very roots. Only then was it recognized that both patients received three times the total dose as planned by the protocol, this despite the queries by the pharmacist and the nurse.

■ ■ ■

One day a surgical friend of mine called and said, "Steve, I need to apologize. I have tarnished the reputation of the hospital."

"Nonsense," I said, "how could you do that?"

"I operated on the wrong side!" he exclaimed.

He had been caring for a weekend warrior athlete with a shoulder problem. The surgeon determined that it would be useful to do arthroscopy— make a small incision and look around inside for torn tissue to repair. The surgeon was widely recognized as excellent, which gave his patient much comfort. The surgery was described as routine, and he would be home the same day. During the procedure the surgeon saw that the joint did not look damaged; the torn cartilage he anticipated wasn't there. Now the light bulb went off, and he realized he was operating on the wrong side. This had never happened to him before; he always took great pains to be sure that everything was set up correctly at the start of surgery. How could he make such a mistake; indeed, why did not the nurses or others point out that he was starting to operate on the wrong side?

■ ■ ■

A small child was brought to the emergency room of a children's hospital in a major metropolitan area. The child had severe pain and a dose of 0.5 mg of morphine was ordered and administered intravenously and then repeated later. The child died because the person drawing up the syringe of morphine mistakenly read the dose as 5.0 mg. A tragedy resulted from a misread decimal point. Should we call this "death by decimal point"?

▪ ▪ ▪

A forty-seven-year-old woman woke up one morning with severe hip pain. She could hardly get out of bed and essentially could not walk. Her orthopedic surgeon diagnosed a slipped disk in her lower back and ordered bed rest and narcotic painkillers to see if the problem would subside without the need for surgery. Over a few days the pain began to recede, but now she had a new problem—constipation. Every reader has had constipation at some time or another, but this was constipation with a capital "C." She was frankly miserable and now needed multiple stool softeners, laxatives, enemas, and a disimpaction (a euphemism for inserting a gloved finger and breaking up the very hard stool in the lower rectum. This sort of task usually is relegated to a medical student or intern when this occurs in the hospital). Why the constipation? Because all narcotics slow down bowel function. Essentially every person given a narcotic for any length of time, especially if bedridden as well, needs a stool softener and laxative. Her doctor forgot to prescribe them.

▪ ▪ ▪

A gentleman was admitted by his internist for abdominal pain; the workup led to surgery. All went well, but a week later the man was running a fever, coughing, and his internist heard sounds in the chest that suggested pneumonia. The doctor told the nurse that he wanted a chest X-ray to confirm his diagnosis and would write an order for an antibiotic. He visited a few other patients and returned to the nurses' station to write the order. But the chart was gone because it was with the patient in the radiology department, so he asked for a blank order sheet. The clerk carefully stamped it with the patient's name and information and the physician wrote an order for an antibiotic from the penicillin family.

Had the chart been present he would have been reminded by the bright red tape on the cover: "Allergic to Penicillin." He had taken that history just a week before but did not recall it just now while writing the order. The failsafe mechanism was thwarted because the chart was not present. Hopefully, the nurse noted the problem before administering the drug and called the physician for a revised drug order.

▪ ▪ ▪

An elderly lady had urinary frequency and some incontinence for a number of years. She used a disposable diaper to ensure that she wouldn't have an accident while out shopping or visiting friends. A gynecologist in the large city about a hundred miles from home had become recognized for a surgical procedure that corrects this problem. She was scheduled to come to the hospital at 6:30 in the morning to be prepared for a 7:30 OR start. She and her husband arranged for their pets to be cared for by a neighbor and drove to the city where they stayed in a hotel the night before the operation. Their son and daughter-in-law had planned time off from their jobs and arranged for their two children to be out of school so that they could fly in from the coast to be with his parents for the first week after the patient returned home.

All was set to go, the patient had been anesthetized and the surgeon was ready to start. But the special instrument that he uses for this operation was not present. A frantic search began in Central Sterile Supply. It could not be found. Finally, an enterprising nurse located one at the other major academic teaching hospital in the city. A cab was sent with a technician to get the instrument and bring it back. It still had to be sterilized. Remarkably, given the frenzied yet effective efforts of many staff members, this lady actually had her surgery that day; she and her husband's time and expense of travel to the city and stay in a hotel were not in vain, and the children's plans to take a leave from work did not have to be changed.

But it could have been different. The surgery could have been called off, the patient sent back home for another time, with all the frustrations and complications that would have ensued as a result. As it was, she was asleep two hours longer than anticipated, which increased the risks for infection and other complications.

HOW FREQUENT ARE PREVENTABLE MEDICAL ERRORS?

These are just some of the stories about errors that I am aware of, some from my own hospital, some from others. But are they the exception to the rule? Or are they commonplace? A study from Harvard Medical School published in the prestigious *New England Journal of Medicine* in 1991, by Lucian Leape, MD, and colleagues, found that operative complications occurred in about 2 percent of all hospitalized patients; just under 1 percent had a drug-related problem, and a total of nearly 4 percent of all patients had some injury secondary to hospital activities.[1]

Another study of errors by Andrews and colleagues, published in the major British journal *The Lancet*, followed 1,047 hospitalized patients on two intensive care units and one surgical floor. They noted that the average patient suffered about 4.5 adverse events during hospitalization, but the range was great—one patient had a total of 52 events! Not surprisingly, those with one or more adverse events spent more time in the hospital (twenty-four days) than those with no events (nine days.)[2]

Data from the American Hospital Association and analyzed by the Healthcare Advisory Board showed 17 to 30 percent of patients had one or more serious events. Convert this to a typical 350-bed community hospital with about 14,000 admissions and 5,400 surgeries, and 4,000 serious adverse events will happen each year.

In this hypothetical American hospital, 884 patients will have an adverse drug event, 816 a *nosocomial infection* (an infection acquired in the hospital), 696 a procedural complication, 544 an unplanned readmission, and 408 a decubitus ulcer; 299 will die; 204 will have a fall, and 163 will have an anesthesia complication.[3]

The message: Adverse events are commonplace, and many, if not most, are preventable.

THE INSTITUTE OF MEDICINE REPORT—TO ERR IS HUMAN

The Institute of Medicine (IOM), in a landmark publication in 1999, wrote that as many as forty-four thousand to ninety-eight thousand Americans die as the result of *preventable* errors in American hospitals each year.[4] These are incredible numbers, and many have disputed them. But even if only half or 10 percent occur, that is way too many. Some studies, however, suggest that the IOM estimates are too low. The IOM report was entitled "To Err Is Human," an apropos title since that is the basic problem. Humans make mistakes. Humans will continue to make mistakes. Well-educated and well-trained humans will make mistakes. Humans that double-check will still make mistakes.

The IOM report noted that deaths from medical mistakes surpassed those from AIDS, breast cancer, or auto accidents. Medication errors were most common; surgery-related errors were the second most common type of error that led to death. The report urged recognition of performance limitations; creation of systems to report errors and near misses; creation of a safety culture; and safety curriculum, team training, and simulation.

It's been seven years since the publication of the IOM report, and much has been said and written. Indeed, many hospitals have started to reduce error rates. But errors still abound, and not nearly enough has been done to make a real and lasting dent, much less to truly drive them down toward zero. Beginning with boards of trustees, little attention is focused on safety; rather it is focused on the financial status of the hospital. Most improvements to date have been the result of mandates, principally from the Joint Commission on Accreditation of Healthcare Organizations (JCAHO). It is time for America's hospital leaders and especially trustees to insist that appropriate changes be made.[5, 6] In this chapter, I will review what needs to be done and suggest specific actions.

HOSPITAL CULTURE AND HOW IT NEEDS TO CHANGE

Unfortunately, the usual hospital culture is one of chastisement and punishment of the culprit: if we make it clear that we will not tolerate such mistakes, certainly people will be more careful. Nothing could be further from the truth, and such a culture encourages covering up and not reporting errors. No one wants to be labeled as inferior; no one wants a letter of reprimand in his or her personnel file or medical staff office. A professional needs to maintain his license to practice. Will an error jeopardize that?

The cure is *not* to punish those who make mistakes—since we all do—but *to create systems to detect errors, correct errors, and help to prevent errors.* At the same time, we need to foster a culture of openness where errors and near misses are discussed and communication is improved. All of this will require that trustees take the lead and insist that safety is critical and that hospital executives will be evaluated on their performance with safety, not just for financial success.

Modern hospitals are the cathedrals of the modern era. They anchor dynamic civic and financial activity and are extraordinarily complex. Patients are complex as are treatment protocols. The coordination needed between different types of health care providers and their dependence on technology adds to the complexity. Throw in the large volume of information needed for decision making and the residual uncertainty inherent in making medical decisions, and the modern hospital becomes still more complex.

Many patients receive more than ten medications per day, many of which are inherently dangerous. The operating room is the financial engine of most health care facilities and also the source of many of the most published adverse events. Nosocomial infections are all too often the result of physician and staff error in performing well-established procedures.

In order to improve safety, the hospital must first create a culture of safety, and then design patient safety initiatives that take into account technology upgrades and human factors. The culture of safety must include an institutional commitment from the board and CEO to adopt appropriate systems and provide required resources of people, time, and dollars. The culture of safety requires a nonpunitive attitude toward medical errors and open communication about errors so that near-miss data can be collected and analyzed to find the root cause of the errors. Accountability must start with the CEO and spread on down through the ranks of physicians and staff to reinforce the desired behaviors.

Human factors that can improve safety include effectively enhancing leadership and management of each hospital unit, improving communication and information transfer, and enhancing training. Using an effective system, such as crew resource management to improve teamwork and align performance measures, reward, and recognition systems, will reinforce the desired changes in both the process and the individuals' behavior.

Process changes, constant checking to improve them, and rigorous adherence to following them, are critical to improving safety. Patient identification, medication administration, infection control, operative standards, and information/communication all need to be considered a process, require agreement, and require subsequent adherence.

Highly reliable organizations become that way because of constant vigilance and continued improvement of processes by testing, auditing, drilling, creating redundancies, and building accountability into everyone's role—regardless of individual preferences.[7]

Once the culture and the human factors have been addressed, multiple technologies can dramatically enhance safety. But it is essential that the culture and human factors are addressed first. Technologies without the needed underlying culture will not be of much help.

The areas to address first with systems changes are medication errors (including blood product administration), operating room and related perioperative events, and hospital acquired infections. In the process, it makes good sense to assure that

- hospitals and their surgical and medical staff only do procedures that they do in large numbers (experience counts)
- intensive care units are staffed by those trained in intensive care medicine (intensivists, not generalists)
- resident physician-trainees are closely supervised (trainees are just that)

LESSONS FROM OTHER INDUSTRIES

Other industries where safety is of utmost concern are the airlines and nuclear power plants. In these industries, safety is the number one priority and is reflected in all leadership and staff performance measures, reward structures, and accountability systems. The organization and culture are designed to get safety to happen. A culture of safety is common to these industries where the inherent risk is acknowledged; a nonpunitive environment encourages error reporting, and recognizing errors is seen as an opportunity to reduce risk; and management commits to structures that reduce risk. Errors are analyzed by root cause and improvements designed into systems to prevent recurrence.

These industries respect human limits and avoid reliance on memory. They use forcing functions and constraints as primary methods rather than education and training as the prime methods to reduce risk. They also have an integrated, highly intensive, and accountable skill indoctrination process for the new employee and regularly scheduled refreshers for existing employees. Team functioning is enhanced, and standardization is the byword.

These industries have developed a culture where attitudes and behaviors are reinforced and a commitment to safety is above efficiency. This includes a provision of the needed resources and openness about errors. The processes end to end, the people system from entry to exit, the information, technology, and the accountability system are all designed together to get safety to be the norm and the culture. The result is industries with stellar safety records.[8, 9]

This is not the way most hospitals do business; it is not their culture. But it needs to be.

MEDICATION ERRORS

Much attention must be given to medication errors since they are the most frequent errors in the hospital. The process of medication delivery has three separate components, each with multiple subcomponents. First, the physician orders a drug for a patient; then the pharmacy processes the order; and finally, the nurse administers the drug. In actual practice, many steps and multiple checks and balances hve been inserted to assure that errors do not occur.

THE CURRENT PROCESS IN MOST HOSPITALS

Ordering. Physicians are famous for poor handwriting. Whether or not the injunction is true, lack of legibility accounts for a large number of errors or, at least, the need to check with the physician for clarity. In some hospitals, the doctors' orders are transcribed by a clerk for transmittal to the pharmacy. The clerk may be careful but is not trained in drug therapy, so an error from misreading handwriting is easily possible.

Since the advent of fax machines, many hospitals have the clerk fax the order directly to the pharmacy; this is quick and eliminates the chance that the clerk will make an error in transcription. Whichever system is used, a nurse is to cross-check the transcription before it is sent off, but this doesn't always happen during busy times, or the nurse may misread the handwriting.

Some 60 percent of all medication errors occur as a result of physician mistake or someone else misreading the order. At my hospital, we observed all orders for a month. A remarkable 42 percent needed some level of remediation before the medication could be filled! Sometimes the nurse or pharmacist asked the physician a simple question, but other times they questioned the dosage or the possibility of an allergic reaction. Often there was no error; but it was still worth checking. Think of the time wasted because the order was not correct, clear, or legible from the start. The good news here, of course, is that the system in place empowered both nurse and pharmacist to double-check the doctor's order.

Preparation in the Pharmacy. Today's hospital pharmacy includes many checks and balances to assure safety, but mistakes still occur. It is not uncommon for the pharmacist to have difficulty interpreting the order. I went to the pharmacy when I was the hospital CEO and asked the director how often they got orders that were difficult to read? "Very frequently," was the answer.

"May I see an example?" I asked.

"Well, let's just go to the inbox and see what's there," he responded.

The first order in the pile was a disaster waiting to happen. I could not read it, at least, not at first. After some time, I figured out that it was a set of drug orders for a patient who was getting a kidney transplant. These powerful drugs could easily be toxic if not given properly. "Will you call the doctor to get this clarified?" I asked.

"No, we do a lot of kidney transplants here, so we know the routine, and we are used to this physician's handwriting, so we can manage with this one."

Wow, I thought. But often they cannot read an order, and this leads to calls and pages. But if the doctor doesn't answer immediately and the drug is needed in a hurry or if the pharmacist thinks he understands the order, it may be prepared and sent to the floor.

Many drugs today come from the manufacturer prepackaged in what are called *unit doses* or packets that are consistent with common prescribing practices. This eliminates error in measuring liquids. You are familiar with those little tubs of cream cheese that are served today in restaurants. For the restaurant this reduces waste and assures that the product is clean when served. Same idea for the pharmacy.

Unit doses of various liquid drugs are arranged alphabetically in the pharmacy bins. Imagine that the physician orders metachlopramide for a patient, three times per day. The pharmacist goes to that bin and pulls out three containers, checks the labels, and puts them in a tray that will go to the patient's floor. Unfortunately, many of these packets look alike and are easy to mistake. Imagine that the patient gets the packet from the next bin by mistake—milk of magnesia. After three doses of that today, he will be an unhappy camper tomorrow! Not the worst of errors, but still a problem.

Other drugs must be placed into an intravenous solution. This requires taking the drug from the shelf in its vial, inserting a needle on a syringe to withdraw the correct amount, then injecting the drug into the intravenous fluid in a bag. But the same drug comes in various concentrations—a frequent cause of error. A pharmaceutical manufacturer wants to have all of its packaging look alike—their "brand." But a look-alike package is potentially deadly if a higher concentration is pulled off the shelf by mistake; an equal amount of fluid removed from the vial might mean a dangerous or even fatal dose into the intravenous bag.

One approach on medical floors is simply to not allow high or dangerous concentrations of drugs on the floor where less-trained but enthusiastic staff might make a mistake. For example, high concentrations of potassium, if not diluted properly, can cause the heart to stop when given intravenously. So it is best to not have the high concentration vials around where someone might misread the label. This simple step has meant big reductions in this error that, unfortunately, was not all that rare.

Pills are often also packaged in "unit of use" plastic bags with a label. The pharmacist can then select the proper pills for a patient without having to open and count from a large container each time. Alternatively, the pill is prepackaged in individual blister packs by the manufacturer and comes with a label noting name and strength. The packaged pills or capsules are placed in bins just like the unit doses of liquids noted above. Of course, the same errors can occur. Consider two pills that look a lot alike. It is all too easy to select the wrong package. Yes, they each have a label, but sometimes the eye does not see the difference. Here is an example of my own with a community pharmacy.

For more than twenty-five years, I cared for a patient who took multiple medications including Xanax (aprazolam) for her anxiety. One day she called and said that she felt terrible. In the office, she seemed dehydrated for no apparent reason. She was admitted, placed on her usual medications, and given intravenous fluids. By the next day, she felt quite good. But we had no idea what had happened. She went back home but called the next day to say that it was starting all over again. After asking her some questions, she said that she was concerned about her Xanax.

"With all these generic drugs, every time I get a refill, the pills look different. Remember those water pills you gave me after my heart attack? The Xanax I picked up last week at the pharmacy looked just like them. But I figured it was just a new generic version of the Xanax."

I had her drive over with her pills and guess what? They were indeed the same diuretic ("water pills") that she had taken some years before. No wonder she was dehydrated! The pharmacist had pulled the wrong pills off the shelf and dispensed them as aprazolam. She had wondered about them, but didn't feel comfortable challenging the pharmacist.

Delivery to the Floor and Administration of Medications. Let's go back to our hospital discussion. The prepared drugs are delivered by the pharmacy to the individual floors or units in the hospital. Each patient has a tray or drawer in a chest that is stationed in the hallway near where the nurse is working. All of Mr. Miller's medications are in that tray, Mrs. Greene's are in another tray, and so on. The tray may be divided into front and rear compartments to separate what he is definitely to be given today and what he may have if he wishes or needs (for example, a sleeping pill or pain medication).

The nurse is expected to check her medication order card and select the proper medications from the tray. Her medication card also notifies her about any allergies or other potential medication issues. She will double-check this against the drugs that she is about to administer to be sure that nothing will cause a problem. Her medication card also indicates the dose and route as transcribed from the physician's order. If anything doesn't match up, she will double-check the original doctor's order or call the physician if she has a question or concern. Once checked, she takes the medicine to the patient and then marks down that it was given. Depending on the patient and the drug, she may stay with the patient to actually see him take it. At the end of the day or shift, nothing should be left in the front half of the tray. All of these steps are set up to assist with patient safety related to medications.

But errors can still occur. A drug gets into the wrong tray, or the nurse opens the wrong tray to take out a medication. It looks correct, and it is given. Or the nurse misses the fact that the patient is known to be allergic, just as the doctor did when signing the original order. Or something has happened to the patient's kidneys, and the original order is no longer appropriate, but the adjustment has not yet been ordered. Will the nurse know or not?

I have a personal story on this issue. Some years ago, my mother fell and broke her hip. She was admitted to her local hospital, about forty miles from where we lived, and an orthopedist was summoned. When I learned about her admission, I called some orthopedic friends to check on the surgeon; he got good marks, and I was relieved. The next day, she was to have her surgery to repair the fracture. My father and I sat in her room with her. Soon the nurse came in with a pre-op antibiotic. "Ampicillin," she said as she injected it into the intravenous line.

I almost had a cardiac arrest. My mother thought she was allergic to penicillin and had told the doctor and nurse. It was written in large red letters on a strip across the front of her chart—I had seen it at the nurses' station a half hour earlier. Ampicillin is a close cousin of penicillin. If you are allergic to penicillin, then you are almost always allergic to ampicillin. Yet my mother had just been given an intravenous dose of ampicillin! Trying to act calmly in front of my mother and father, I pointed out my mother's presumed allergy and suggested that the nurse prepare for a reaction.

Fortunately, she was not really allergic, as the next few minutes would testify. What went wrong? The doctor was in the OR and had called with his order for ampicillin; he did not remember that she was presumably allergic, and the nurse did not make the association that allergy to penicillin is to be treated like allergy to ampicillin. (Ampicillin was not a good choice of prophylaxis for hip surgery anyway . . . another story for another time.)

What can be done to reduce these errors? Humans will still make mistakes, so just more training and admonitions to be careful are not enough. The various checks and balances built in now are good, but not good enough. A new way of approaching medications includes the use of various technologies to keep health care practitioners from making mistakes and ensure that any mistakes that are made are caught before they harm the patient.

PROPOSED FUTURE PROCESS

Ordering. The physician does all ordering via computer.

The physician signs in with name and password and then scrolls to the patient's record. Only the appropriate physician has access to actually creating or changing a medication order for this particular patient. Others can see the order but cannot make changes. The physician now prescribes the medication, including dose, route, and number of times per day. The computer will query the reason for the order.

Take for example an antibiotic given for pneumonia. If the patient is known to be allergic, the computer will not accept the order. If the dose is inappropriate for the patient's height and weight, it will challenge the order or assist the physician in calculating the correct dose. If the patient's kidneys are malfunctioning (known to the computer because the blood tests of kidney function are also incorporated into the system), it will alert the physician to adjust the dose and, again, assist in that calculation. If the patient is receiving other drugs that might interact adversely with the new drug, the computer will so inform the physician. If the antibiotic chosen for pneumonia is not among those usually used for pneumonia, the computer will also query the doctor, even suggesting alternatives. All of these steps will be instantaneous and convenient. We could call this *Alerts and Built-in Knowledge* in the computer software.

There are some problems. First, these are new systems, and they are constantly being updated and upgraded. The basics work well, but the added elements are still coming. Clearly, such a system eliminates the handwriting error. It eliminates the allergy error. So mistakes will be much lessened. By adding "knowledge" such as drug-drug interaction, kidney function, and choice of antibiotic, the physician is given additional help and is taught all at the same time. The training comes at the perfect moment. Doctors learn best when faced with an issue, such as determining the best antibiotic to prescribe right now for pneumonia, not when the doctor is reading about pneumonias at home, from a textbook.

Drug Preparation in the Pharmacy. If a physician uses the computer to write an order, there is no chance for misreading handwriting. That is a big first step that reduces errors immensely. The pharmacist can review the order and see how it has been adjusted for kidney function, other drugs being administered, and dosed for weight and height. The computer can set up alerts and alarms to the pharmacist for any order that was sent despite the computer's advice. The pharmacist does not have to enter the order into the pharmacy computer; it is done automatically.

Drugs can be selected from the bins described previously and then scanned with a bar code just as in the supermarket. This not only records that the drug was placed in the patient's tray but it cross-checks the selection. Is it the right drug, right dose, right number of doses for the day? If the pharmacist or pharmacy technician selects a higher concentration of the drug, the bar code reader alerts the computer, which in turn stops the process. This will dramatically decrease the chance for taking dangerous concentrations of a drug and mistakenly under- or over-diluting it for addition to intravenous fluid. Further, the computer, having checked the concentration of the drug in the vial and knowing what is needed to add to the IV solution, now prompts the pharmacy technician with the correct amount to withdraw.

Pills, capsules, and liquids packaged in unit doses or units of use can be stored and retrieved by a pharmacy robot. The robot is given directions by the computer that in turn is following the doctor's orders, as checked and verified by the pharmacist. The robot selects the ordered drugs, checks its bar code, and delivers it to the patient's tray. Basically, the robot has a special arm that grasps the package and moves it to the tray.

The process actually starts by having the robot stock a location with multiple sets of the bar coded, prepackaged drug. The robot knows the location and will return there when it needs that drug for a patient. But it still double-checks by reading the bar code on the drug package before proceeding. If somehow a drug gets into the wrong location, the robot will pick it up and put it into a discard tray.

Delivery to the Floor and Administration of Medications. Another new step in protecting the patient is a special distribution cart or case on the hospital unit floor. Instead of a cart with many drawers or trays that can be opened by anyone, multiple features are built into the new system. First, the robot or pharmacy technician loads the cart with the various patients' trays. The cart is connected with the computer that knows the patient's orders and what the pharmacy has prepared.

The nurse goes to the cart but cannot open it. Instead, she or he must first sign in with name and password and then the specific patient's name. A nurse from elsewhere in the hospital, not assigned to that floor, will not have access to this cart. Next, the nurse indicates which drug she wishes to withdraw. The computer and nurse co-verify the choice and the patient's drawer (and only that patient's drawer) opens automatically. The nurse removes the desired medication, and then swipes it across the bar code reader on the cart to verify both that it is correct and that it was removed.

The nurse then goes to the patient's room, swipes the patient's bar code enhanced wrist identification band, and gets an approval from her computer—handheld or on a movable cart—which is, in turn, connected wirelessly to the hospital clinical information system, including the medication-ordering software.

Once the approval is posted, the drug is given and the system registers the transaction as completed, eliminating that paperwork from the nurse's routine.

From end to end, the order is checked continuously: a record of who was involved (doctor, pharmacist, pharmacy technician, nurse); a continuous record of any changes made, why and by whom and with whose approval; assurance that the right drug got to the right patient at the right time in the correct dosage and route; and a record of when the medication was actually administered or swallowed. In addition, if mistakes were made and the computer issued a correction or alert, it will be recorded as well.

The latter is an interesting issue. Consistent with the airline pilots' agreement to report errors and near misses with the promise of anonymity, it might be best to keep this data unconnected with the individuals involved. This will encourage physicians, nurses, and pharmacists to use the computerized system without fear of reprisals for making an error. Yet the institution can collect valuable data to analyze, so that the system can change in response to common or recurrent errors. Of course it would also be valuable to learn that a particular doctor repeatedly made the same mistake. In this instance, he or she could be offered some form of remediation, but this would break the anonymity. A balance will be needed.

HOSPITAL-ACQUIRED INFECTIONS

Surgery-Associated Infections: Slightly less than 3 percent of all operations result in a surgically associated infection. That represents about 780,000 such infections each year in U.S. hospitals. Infections increase the risk of death during the hospitalization, obviously increase discomfort, increase the length of hospital stay, and increase the cost of the hospitalization by about three thousand dollars, often more. Operating room procedures have long stressed sterile conditions. The room is prepped before surgery; all of the instruments are sterilized; the surgeon, scrub tech, and nurses carefully scrub their hands with antiseptic before surgery and don sterile gown and gloves. Still infections occur.

Certain types of surgery benefit from prophylactic antibiotics: open-heart surgery, bowel surgery, surgery associated with trauma. One common problem is that antibiotics administered intravenously at the time of surgery to prevent infection are often not given as indicated. The best time is about twenty minutes before the surgery starts, in other words, twenty minutes before the incision is made. This allows for a high concentration of the drug in the bloodstream during the critical time. But it is not uncommon for the antibiotics to be forgotten, given much later, or too early. Generally this is a problem of "I forgot" because other more apparently critical issues demand action at the time, another example of "to err is human."

Simply chastising the anesthesiologist to remember will likely not help much. The best approach is to create special reminders that prompt the staff to give the antibiotic. A surgical computer information system, loaded with the patient's orders, can automatically create such a prompt and record when the drug is actually administered.

Another simple step that helps is clipping hair, not shaving. For decades the approach was to shave off hair near the incision site. The idea was to get as much of the hair out of the way as possible. But shaving inevitably leads to small nicks that can be the nidus for an infection. Much better to clip. Another problem is for the patient to be cold during surgery. Operating rooms are traditionally kept cool because the bright lights and equipment give off heat, and the surgeons and nurses get too hot to be comfortable inside their sterile gowns and gloves. But a cold patient is a patient at greater risk of infection. A new and simple approach covers the patient with a special blanket that circulates warm air. This, too, has been shown to reduce infection.

Some patients must be kept cool during surgery. For example, body temperature is lowered during open-heart surgery because the heart can better tolerate being stopped for a period if it is cool. Speaking of heart surgery, those with diabetes need to have their blood sugar monitored during surgery. If it should get too high, it increases the risk of a postoperative infection.

Unit-Acquired Infections: Infections occur for many reasons. A surgical wound that does not heal properly may get infected. The site of an intravenous catheter may get infected. A patient with a urinary catheter may get a urinary infection. A patient on a respirator may get infected in the lungs. And patients whose natural defenses against infection are reduced by drugs, such as cancer chemotherapy or antirejection drugs for transplants, are at risk for infection.

Preventing infections is straightforward, if not always so easy. Pay careful attention to the surgical wound after surgery. Remove and replace, if necessary, the intravenous catheters every few days. Limit the time urinary catheters are used. Replace the respirator tubing every few days. But first and foremost, wash your hands before visiting and examining the patient.

A surgeon going into the operating room will wash carefully before donning the sterile gown and gloves for surgery. It is the culture of the OR—a culture that started the first day as a medical or nursing student assigned to the OR. A stern nurse oversaw the washing technique: "Scrub for a full ten minutes." "Use that scrub brush more." "Get under your fingernails." "I'm watching you!" The culture is strong, and no one would break it without fear of instant reproach by all colleagues.

But put that same surgeon on the general hospital floors, visiting patients on rounds, and watch how often he or she washes hands. Not very often. So hospitals have tried many techniques: Put sinks in every room—they are ignored. Put the sink just outside the door to the room—still ignored much of the time. It is the same for internists and pediatricians and all physicians. Nurses are generally much better, but far from perfect. Washing regularly after every patient encounter, for instance, can lead to chapped hands, which is actually worse because more germs can be carried on broken skin.

As a young attending physician in 1973, I decided to study how often the physician team members washed before examining patients on morning rounds at our branch of the National Cancer Institute in Baltimore. First, I spent a two-month period teaching the group about the importance of hand washing, especially as these were cancer patients with vastly deficient body defenses, getting powerful chemotherapy drugs. And I tried to serve as a good role model on rounds, so everyone saw that the attending physician followed what he preached. Then I was on assignment elsewhere for three months. When I returned, I made no further comment while I watched what happened. During the next month, one physician on one occasion washed his hands!

Yet these were smart, dedicated, reliable physicians whose desire for good patient care was paramount in their minds. But hand washing did not seem that important. True, few sinks were available at that time, but even when it was nearby, the sink was rarely used. It just did not seem all that important. The next month, when prompted to wash, each physician dutifully complied. So the problem was not unwillingness, but lack of attention and lack of a strong culture that valued hand washing as essential, a culture in which colleagues would hold one in contempt if the normal routine were not followed. It is simple human behavior, and in order to make the hospital safer, we need to focus on what makes a person behave in the needed fashion.

Not having enough sinks doesn't help, however. And frequent hand washing with soap does dry out your hands. Johnson and Johnson had a product called "Intercept" in the 1970s that appeared to be valuable. It came in a canister the size of a physician's penlight and had a clip so that it could be stored in the doctor's white coat pocket. Pull it out and press the button and a material the consistency of shaving cream emerged. It was made of various antiseptics, including alcohol that killed bacteria on contact. It also had skin creams included so that the alcohol did not dry out your hands. Numerous tests of this product at the Cancer Center showed that it was quite effective at killing germs, had a long-lasting effect, did not damage skin, and was simple to use.

Although I would never suggest only intermittent use to our staff, in fact, their hands stayed relatively germ-free over a prolonged period, even when examining multiple patients without reapplication. Our doctors and nurses were not perfect in using it, but much better than with the sink. Unfortunately, the company withdrew the product because of limited sales. I have often wished I had stocked up while it was still available.

More recently, the basic concept has been revived. Alcohol-based products are on the market and come in various sized plastic bottles or in pump-type canisters. (You may have seen them in restrooms or may have picked up a small container for use while traveling.) These can be placed in the patients' rooms, or they can be attached to the door frame outside each patient's room. The hope is that doctors and nurses will use these simple, quick, nongreasy, and nonirritating products before entering a patient's room. Because they are formulated with hand lotions, they do not chap the skin or dry it out. Time will tell, but early trials have been successful. Still, a culture of attentiveness will be essential before hand washing or hand disinfecting becomes the standard.

The point is that most hospital-acquired infections do not have to occur. They do occur because simple yet effective procedures are not being used, from hand washing by staff to hair clipping at the planned incision site to proper use of prophylactic antibiotics before surgery. Properly followed, these approaches will dramatically reduce infection, which can cause longer hospital stays, increase costs, and even lead to death.

What will it take to make it happen? This is a good place to discuss human behavior analysis. We mostly do what we think others will reward us for or avoid doing what we will be punished for. A simple analogy is speeding. Near where I live, a new highway was completed. It is longer by a mile than the old route to the medical center, but it has no traffic lights whereas the old route has multiple stop-and-go crossroads. The speed limit on the new road is 55 mph, but it is sure easy to go faster, especially when traffic is light. The signs clearly say "55," but many ignore them. So the state troopers patrol regularly and set up speed traps almost daily. They make a real show of stopping speeders, not just to catch the speeder, but also to remind all of us to stick to the posted limit. They are responding to human behavior patterns. Everyone reads the sign that says "55 mph," but it only affects their driving if it is clear that there are consequences, negative consequences, for exceeding the limit.

So, too, in the hospital. Tell me to wash my hands, and I will understand that it is important. But if I also know that my chief of service will get after me if I do not, then I will pay more attention. What we need in the hospital are more "state troopers" in the guise of nursing heads, medical chiefs, and others who insist that the standards be met, all the time, every day. Otherwise, human behavior is such that we will slip. That is the problem in hospitals today. Those in positions of authority do not spend the time and energy to enforce the standards, and this needs to change.

IMPROVING SAFETY IN THE OR AND THROUGHOUT THE HOSPITAL

After I retired, I began to assist the Army in a project addressing safety in the OR. During a recent ten-month period, I interviewed more than one hundred surgeons, anesthesiologists, nurses, and others at multiple academic medical centers across the United States who worked in the OR or the overall *perioperative environment* (the prep area, the recovery room, and all the affiliated areas that support the ORs). Certain common themes emerged. The OR (and by extension, most procedure-based areas of the hospital like the cardiac catheterization laboratory or the gastroenterology suite) is a highly complex, high-velocity, high-stress work site. Communication is generally less than satisfactory, and the professionals involved do not function as a true team. The communication technique called "read back," as practiced in an aircraft or naval bridge ("Air traffic control to UA 122, turn right to 15 degrees" is replied by "UA 122, roger, turn right to 15 degrees"), is simply not part of the medical culture. Nor are checklists, as used by the cockpit crew before every takeoff. Scrub nurses and technicians report that they are discouraged from confronting the attending surgeon when they observe an error or potential error: "We work in the OR as three separate professions, each doing our job, but certainly not acting as a team."

Important OR Issues

- 20% (At Least) Medical Errors Occur in Perioperative Environment
- Patient Asleep (cannot assist in error mitigation)
- High Velocity Environment
- High Complexity Environment
- Or Team Not a True Team
- Communication a Major Issue

No one wants to report errors or near misses. The culture is that "professionals just don't make mistakes," but if one does make an error and it is detected by senior individuals, especially in nursing departments, chances are high the person will be reprimanded or possibly even fired. Further, the nurse who witnesses a mistake or sees a surgeon who is clearly not trained to use a new piece of equipment is loath to report it because she/he has to work with that physician again tomorrow. It's a culture "designed" for failure and exacerbated by the increased pressure from hospital executives to make ever more effective use of these highly expensive facilities.

What can be done? A straightforward, if not easy, four-part program can make substantial strides in improving safety. It includes changing the culture, making error and near-miss reporting standard, addressing teamwork and communication, and engaging certain technologies, such as information systems and simulators. A look at what occurred in the airline industry is illustrative of what can be done.

THE ANALOGY OF THE AIRLINE COCKPIT

An airline cockpit is often compared to an operating room. Although clearly an imperfect analogy, it has merit. The captain is not only the senior pilot, but is also "the captain of the ship" with ultimate responsibility. Until recently, he (rarely she) was looked upon by the first officer and flight engineer or navigator with awe, respect, and fear. *Awe* because the captain had been successful in moving up the ranks to the position of captain, a position the lower-ranked officers aspired to obtain. *Respect* because the captain, indeed, had the years of experience that brought with it much knowledge and skill. But also *fear* because in the hierarchical world of the cockpit, junior officers were to do their work but never question the authority or the wisdom of the captain even if they thought he had made a mistake. To question that authority was to risk a negative report in one's record. This all began to change in the mid-1970s as it became apparent that the vast majority of airline mishaps were the result of pilot error and most specifically to problems in communication related to the culture of the cockpit.

This sounds much like the operating room of today with the attending surgeon the "captain," a position obtained through years of training and experience—a training system that also trained everyone to accept a hierarchical standard of behavior as normal. No resident would question the "chief" because to do so might lead to disparaging words at the least and loss of opportunities for "good" cases in the OR at worst. Scrub nurses and technicians, under the cover of confidentiality, consistently attest to a system with poor communication and limited teamwork because of the current culture of the OR.

The cockpit has changed, and with the change has come a remarkable improvement in airline safety, along with improved morale and reduced turnover of staff. The focus has been on designing a culture that reinforces teamwork, communication, flattening the hierarchy, managing error, situational awareness, and decision making—along with nonpunitive near-miss reporting (more than 500,000 reports in fifteen years). It ensures the positive reinforcement of those who report errors and call a "time out" for safety reasons. Hospitals will only see real improvements to safety when a similar culture change occurs.[9]

Approaches to Improved Patient Safety

- Culture of Safety
- Error Reporting & Analysis
- Human Factors
- Technology Factors

CULTURE OF SAFETY

Every hospital CEO and CFO knows that the OR and the procedure units like the cardiac catheterization laboratory and the GI endoscopy suite are the financial heart of the institution. They also need to learn that this is where errors are most prevalent and dangerous and to invest the time, people, and money to make improvements. Just as we discussed with medication safety, the first step is for the culture of punishment for an error to give way to a nonpunitive culture where step two, reporting incidents, is the norm, and open discussion is cherished.

Whether or not reporting is anonymous, rapid review and root cause analysis with appropriate feedback must happen in a reasonable time frame. Further, the hospital must institute systems based on these analyses that will keep the staff from making the same type of error in the future. In short, the hospital culture must recognize that "to err is human," and it is incumbent upon the institution to assist in preventing or reversing the inevitable human mistake.

The third step is to aggressively institute a program of "crew resource management" that teaches briefings, communication, assertion, cross-checking, verification, and decision making. Each one is a trait that can be improved with appropriate training and practice. This is combined with teamwork training, which emphasizes effective communication, conflict resolution, and collaborative problem solving.

Let's consider briefings as one example. These briefings are meant to be an overview, not a long discussion, which transmits a few key facts related to the work to be done by the team. The briefing sets the tone, discusses the elements of the procedure, and hand-offs that may be expected. It establishes team and individual competence by organizing everyone and focusing on each team member's role in the procedure. When properly conducted it will be "owned" by the entire team and fosters an environment where any team member can speak up if he or she detects a problem. Using briefings and the other techniques of crew resource management, it is possible to reduce errors while improving morale and reducing turnover of nurses and others. In addition, errors that do occur are more often discussed openly.[9]

Finally, the hospital must look at various technologies that can keep the health care professional from making an error.

Computer entry medication orders (as discussed previously), readily accessible digitized medical data, bar coding, or radio frequency (RFID) identification of equipment and instruments can all help. Video recording of procedures allows postprocedure review and analysis. Some physicians will initially object to being filmed, but consider football: every NFL team spends most of Monday reviewing its performance of the day before, looking for preventable errors, procedural deviations, and ways to improve.

Simulators can make a substantial improvement in individual performance. Full-scale simulators such as those used by aircraft pilots are not yet available, but simulators for specific procedures and techniques are. Indeed, when the FDA recently approved a new stent for *carotid* artery stenosis (the large artery that runs through the neck to the brain, which if clogged can cause a stroke), it also mandated that every physician who wishes to insert this stent must first demonstrate competence with the affiliated simulator. The day is not far off when simulators will be ubiquitous for physician practice, and assessment and resident training programs will begin with a simulator rather than with a patient.

In time, robotics may assist in safety as well. Not autonomous robots, but physician-controlled procedural assistants that can compensate for hand tremors; assure precise insertion of a needle, probe, or device into an organ based upon stereotactic principles; or prevent movement of an instrument outside of predefined safety zones.[10]

Such a four-part approach to procedure-based safety will allow for a healthier environment where error can be reported and openly discussed; where improved communication can lead to not only fewer errors, but also improved morale; and where information technology can assist in data capture and presentation, video can allow for procedural review, and simulation will lead to much-improved training and practice. But the first step is for senior hospital executives and physician leaders to recognize that the OR and procedure-based units need sustained, intensive attention to the safety of our patients. With such appropriate attention to the four-part approach proposed here, well-meaning, well-trained, committed medical professionals will be much less likely to inadvertently "crash into a mountain."

SPECIFIC RESPONSES TO THE EXAMPLES AT THE BEGINNING OF THIS CHAPTER

Let's go back to the beginning of this chapter and look again at the cases I described of preventable medical errors.

Feeding tube line inserted into intravenous line in a newborn premature infant. Before I called the board chairman, I wanted to learn more about what happened. So I asked for a quick root cause analysis. Within an hour, I was told that the staffing levels were fine that night, there were no concurrent emergencies or multiple phone calls to distract the nurse. Other staff members were not off on breaks or getting medications. It looked like a straightforward human error without any obvious predisposing factors. The nursing department felt the nurse should be fired because "professionals don't make this type of mistake."

As I mentioned earlier, this was my wake-up call on patient safety. Here are the decisions that were made: Not to fire the nurse. Get her some counseling because she must be devastated at what happened. Make sure that the family is properly informed, apologize sincerely, and make quick financial restitution. Don't dicker. Investigate a more thorough root cause analysis and offer suggestions as to how the hospital could have supported this nurse so that the error could have been avoided.

Here is what followed: The nurses colleagues noted that she was treated as a caring professional rather than a criminal and hence were more likely to assist in searching for appropriate ways to prevent such an error in the future. The methodology to prevent errors of this type proved to be fairly simple. The intravenous tubing and feeding tubing look different, but are still somewhat similar. Henceforth, the feeding tubing would have a blue line running its length making it more obvious. Further, instead of a round male to female junction, the feeding tube would have a triangular junction; it would be essentially impossible to insert the triangular feeding tube into the round intravenous line socket. I asked why we had not done this before if the technology was available. The answer hurt.

"Well, Dr Schimpff, do you remember that cost-saving program that you instituted? These tubes with the blue lines and the triangular junctions cost a lot more. And we just never thought this type of mistake would be made."

So from then on, the new approach was instituted. But I still needed to call the board chairman and tell him that that infant he had marveled at was dead.

Incorrect dose of highly toxic cancer chemotherapy. This episode made national headlines in the early 1990s. Consistent with the tenor of the times, the fellow was reprimanded. Further, the state board of nursing threatened a large number of nurses with licensure removal on the basis that even though the drug was ordered by the physician and carefully reviewed by the pharmacist, it was the nurse's responsibility to ensure that it was the correct dose. The physician-in-chief, a highly respected clinician and researcher, was forced to resign his position; even though he was not personally involved in the event, he was held ultimately responsible. A culture of fear rapidly engulfed the institution. Errors would be punished. But after some reflection and soul-searching, along with analysis of why errors occur in settings like these, the Cancer Center instituted a new approach with a mind-set that systems needed to be in place to assure that such events could not be repeated and to encourage all of the staff to feel comfortable in reporting problems as they occurred.

Operating on the wrong side. The surgeon was mortified by his error, noting that he had never made such a mistake in more than twenty-five years of practice. Like the nurse caring for the premature infant, he needed assistance in recognizing that the error was part of human nature and did not mean that he was no longer a competent surgeon. Today, the systems approach to preventing this type of laterality error is to have the patient, nurse, and surgeon all agree immediately presurgery as to the proper site and to mark it with a pen. Often the surgeon personally "signs" the site before the patient is anesthetized and draped.

Failure to prescribe stool softeners and possible laxative with narcotic. The surgeon in this case was accustomed to working in a hospital setting where others such as residents and nurses would look after the issues of bowel care. In this instance he was doing a friend a favor by treating her in the home setting. He forgot about the tendency for a patient in pain, immobilized in bed, and on narcotics to develop serious constipation. The dispensing pharmacist should always stress the need for bowel care when delivering the narcotic. The label should automatically print out a reminder, just as reminders are put on prescription bottles stating that a drug should be taken with meals—a simple means of assuring that the patient and patient's family are informed.

Allergy to prescribed antibiotic. In this example, the physician knew the patient was allergic to penicillin, but forgot. The usual safety mechanism in the hospital setting is to have a large sticker on the front of the chart that boldly proclaims the allergy. But in this case, the chart had gone with the patient to the X-ray department. Two other fail-safe mechanisms are built into the hospital system. First, the nurse usually reviews the order before it is sent to the pharmacy, but in this case, the chart was still off the floor, so again the allergy was missed. Second, when the drug is sent to the floor, the administering nurse has a card on the medication cart that lists the patient's medications and also notes any allergies. This notation is a compilation of the admitting nurse's own history from the patient and the physician's note on allergies. Normally, this notation will be sufficient to block the drug from being given. But, occasionally, it happens anyway.

This case is ideal to reiterate the total system for medication error reduction I presented earlier. It begins with the physician's computer order entry. The computer will immediately tell the physician that the patient is allergic to penicillin-like drugs and block the order. That prevents the mistake. But the information system can also add knowledge or training by prompting the physician that for a hospital-acquired pneumonia, the drug he's chosen is not the most effective. It might note that his infectious disease colleagues would generally recommend one of the following three drugs for this situation.

Here the physician will get a quick remedial education on hospital-acquired pneumonia, including the current most appropriate drugs to consider. The computer will also help him adjust the dosage if the patient's kidney function is reduced or suggest alternatives if the antibiotic could possibly interact with another medication the patient is already receiving. Finally, it will create prompts to remind the physician days later that the patient has now had what would usually be a sufficient course of the antibiotic.

Once the order is complete, it will transmit electronically to the pharmacy where it will be reviewed by the pharmacist with the help of a pharmacy information system. This system will double-check dosing, drug-drug interactions, and appropriateness of the drug for this indication. The system will then assist the pharmacy technician in preparing the medication if it requires mixing, or it will direct the pharmacy robot to collect the medication and place it in the specially marked tray for this specific patient.

On the floor, the nurse will check the wireless computer monitor near the bedside, enter her name and password and the patient's name, and the drawer to the medication cabinet assigned to this patient will open. She will take out the marked drug, swipe it with the bar code reader to be sure it is correct and go to the bedside. There she will again swipe the barcode on the drug and the barcode on the patient's wrist. If everything matches, she will administer the drug, and the computer will automatically record it as completed.

All of this will save a great amount of time for the doctor, pharmacist, and nurse; provide a safer environment, and ensure that not only is the drug correct, but also that it is the best drug for that indication. In the process, it helps a number of people in the chain of drug delivery to avoid the natural tendency to make an error. Unfortunately, only a few hospitals have these systems installed, but I predict that they will become the norm during the next five to ten years. And the embedded "knowledge" will be many times better than what I just described.

Missing instrument in the operating room. The critical instrument was missing, leading to a rushed search and, ultimately, the need to borrow a similar one from another hospital. The case was prolonged while all this happened but easily could have resulted in a canceled operation, a frustrated surgeon, and an angry patient, spouse, and family who had spent money not covered by insurance to travel to the city, arrange for pet care, take leave from work and school, and fly home to help take care of Mom after surgery.

This type of error occurs all too often in today's operating room. Information technology and associated technologies are the essential ingredients to improve patient safety and OR efficiency together. The "fix" is to have systems in place to ensure that all equipment and instruments are ready, that the schedule is logical for the cases at hand, that staffing is available for all cases, and that a backup plan is in place should an emergent or urgent case need to be inserted into the schedule. In addition, RFID tags on instruments and equipment can keep track of where key items are located, so that it will be clear in advance when a critical instrument is missing—even where it can be found. Such surgical information systems are just coming into use at a few institutions, and RFID technologies are under study at a few hospitals. Here again, I predict that these systems will be commonplace in time, but it may take ten to fifteen years.

Wrong dose of narcotic given as a result of misreading a decimal point. This is a common mistake in drug preparation. Often numbers are hard to read, sometimes because the mind just sees the dose expected (5.0 mg is a common amount to give an adult; 0.5 mg seems incorrect and is converted to what the mind expects to see). Here again, computer order entry will assist. Because the child was in the ER, the computer may not know the child's weight, but its age would be known from the moment of arrival. Armed with this information, the computer would reject an order of 5.0 mg for this infant and would block the pharmacist from seeing the dosage incorrectly.

MEGATRENDS RELATED TO PATIENT SAFETY

Safety is becoming recognized as important yet is still underappreciated and way underfunded. First, I predict that boards of trustees will finally recognize their responsibility and their critical role in reducing errors in the hospital. From this will come appropriate accountability measures throughout, beginning with the CEO, based on classic human behavior patterns. For example, "You are being measured and rewarded (or not) based on the level of safety in our hospital." Second, basic straightforward approaches will improve safety. Changing the culture to a nonpunitive one with error reporting and analysis is coming—but slowly. The use of crew resource management is effective but still rarely used in most hospitals, but its day will come.

Third, some exciting new developing technologies can markedly assist in reducing errors. Improvements in the electronic medical record, video technologies, RFID, and bar coding will be of major assistance in the years to come. Computer entry of orders by physicians, pharmacy robots, and bar coding all medications will have a positive impact. I believe the really big technology breakthrough will be simulators. They will fundamentally change the approach to training physicians and other health care providers. No longer will it be "see one, do one, teach one." It will be "practice on the simulator until you are deemed competent." Then, and only then, will you be allowed to do it under supervision on a patient. And finally, robotics will add a level of accuracy that the human hand and eye cannot. Fourth and perhaps most important, patients will demand safe environments, and regulators like the JCAHO will continue to insist on adoption of methods like those we have reviewed here.

THE MEGATRENDS

- Trustees Will Take Charge
- Accountability Systems Based On Human Behavior Analysis Will Appear
- Crew Resource Management Will Be Introduced
- Technologies Will Become Commonplace
  - Electronic Drug Ordering & Electronic Medical Record
  - Pharmacy Robots
  - RFID and Bar Coding
  - Video
  - Simulators
  - Surgical Robots
- Regulation And Patient Insistence Will Push the System

WHAT YOU SHOULD KNOW

The key lesson or take-away is that errors occur and will continue to occur no matter how intelligent, caring, or committed your physician, nurse, or pharmacist is. They, like you, are human and humans are prone to error. Rather than look at errors as something in need of punishment, we need to look at errors as something to discuss and understand. Then we need to set up mechanisms to assist well-intentioned practitioners from either committing an error or recognizing it before it can cause harm. Hospitals are large complicated places so a culture of safety is needed, beginning with the board of trustees and CEO, and then throughout the professional staff. Some straightforward techniques can help us overcome our human tendencies toward error and some developing technologies will help to reduce errors.

I predict that people like you will demand that their hospital attend to these issues, not as an afterthought but as a primary responsibility. It will take effort, time, and many resources, but it is clear that the opportunity is rich to markedly reduce errors and harm to patients. This is a hospital's and its staff's greatest obligation to you, its patient and customer.

WHAT YOU CAN DO

What if you need to be admitted to a hospital? First, remember that you have a choice. It is your health and your health care; you are the customer, and you can go elsewhere. So if you need surgery, find out if the surgeon who has been recommended does a lot of the type of surgery that you need. And what is his record of success? Complication rates? Some types of surgery are fairly common, so the surgeon should have a track record that you can ask about.

Sometimes it may be uncommon surgery, but then you still want to know that your surgeon is the one in the region who does the procedure the most often, on a relative basis. Need a colonoscopy? Ask how many the gastroenterologist has done and ask what sort of complication rate does he or she have. Ever cause a perforation? Any other problems? You should feel free to ask. Actually, the physician should offer this information to you from the start.

It is a good idea to have someone with you while you are in the hospital or while being evaluated. You are anxious, possibly even outright scared. A friend or loved one can help write down information relayed by the doctors and nurses. All too often we forget what we were told because so much is going on in our minds at a time of stress, which is just what being in the hospital is—stress! Also, write down your questions so that when the doctor or nurse comes by, you can ask them without forgetting something.

When the nurse brings you a pill, ask what pill it is and what it is for. Remember that you are about to swallow it, so it is important to check. And if a medication is given by vein, ask about it as well. If it is a medicine that your doctor did not tell you about, refuse it! There is no excuse for your physician not to tell you what is being ordered for you and why. It is your health care, not the doctor's.

The same thing goes for a test or procedure. "We are taking you to X-ray for a PET scan that your doctor ordered" is not satisfactory, unless you know why the doctor wanted you to have it. In short, you need to become your own best advocate—and to use your companion as another advocate to check on what is happening and why.

These are all things that you can do directly to help ensure safety. But you can also ask about what your hospital does about collecting error reports. Does a group do root cause analysis? Once patterns are recognized, are changes instituted? Is there a safety agenda, and do the trustees get involved— really involved? If you are having, say, open-heart surgery, is this a hospital where a lot of these cases are done, and not just by your surgeon? In other words, does the staff have a strong level of knowledge and expertise related to this procedure?

What if I must be placed in an intensive care unit, will I be cared for by board-certified intensivists or by my regular doctor? (You know and respect your own doctor, but ICUs are complex places, and your care is best managed by an expert in intensive care medicine.) And is an intensivist available twenty-four hours a day? (Problems occur as often or more often at night and on weekends as during the weekday.) And does this hospital have a computer-based system for the doctors to order medications? And if so, does it include checks on allergies, drug dosage, and drug interactions? What about bar-coded medications and blood transfusions?

Maybe this seems like a lot of questions to ask, and I guess it is. But my purpose is to try to encourage you to take a proactive role in your hospitaliza-tion. You are very important to you and your loved ones. You are important to the doctors and nurses as well; they do not want you to suffer a mishap. But you need to look out for number one, and these are some of the questions that will help you do that in a nonthreatening but informed manner. Not only that, but when more and more people start to ask these questions, hospital staff will become even more attuned to the needs for safe practice.

CHAPTER 11

It's Your Body—Keep It Healthy

So far, we have talked about the various megatrends occurring in medicine that will impact medical care during the next five to fifteen years. Let's think about them briefly from the perspective of a few of the major diseases that cause death or disability. A good place to start is with heart disease. As we look forward to the next five to fifteen years, I predict that open-heart surgery will become less and less common.

Angioplasty and stents, especially biodegradable stents with built-in drugs to prevent reocclusion of the arteries, will be better and better and will result in fewer coronary artery bypass graft operations. Even more important will be new ways to clean out the coronary arteries, kind of like a Roto-Rooter cleansing. Then the cleaned-out arteries will be naturally relined with normal vessel cells, possibly imported as a form of stem cell. The commonly used diagnostic catheterization will become a rarity. Instead, the coronary arteries and the rest of the heart will be imaged with CT scans, MRI scans, or ultrasound giving exquisite anatomical detail tied to a precise measure of their function.

Indeed, heart function overall will be evaluated with these same technologies as well as PET scanning and other developing molecular imaging techniques. Muscle repair following a heart attack will become a reality. Stem cells will be mobilized and directed to the damaged areas for prompt repair. For those who do have major damage to their heart muscle leading to heart failure, the opportunity for a heart transplant will be immediate—without an interminable wait, a mechanical device to tide them over, or death during the wait. And there will be no need for antirejection drugs and all their toxicities—the transplanted heart will come from a pig.

As regards to cancer, today's extensive surgery, intensive radiation therapy, and toxic chemotherapy will be remembered as barbaric. Prevention will become a reality as genomics gives advanced warning and recommends preventive approaches. Cancer will be diagnosed early when just a few cancer cells are present. Therapy will be specific—designed to kill cancer cells, and only cancer cells, without significant side effects. And these specific therapies will be aimed at the originators of the cancer—the cancer stem cells that keep the cancer growing. Genomics will classify cancers not by their anatomy but by their root cause, and this will direct new diagnostic methods and specific targeted therapeutic approaches. Cancer will become, at worst, a chronic disease and many, many more cases will be prevented overall. Those that aren't will be detected early and cured.

As we enter an era of diabetes mellitus occurring in epidemic proportions, many new approaches to treatment will emerge. Newer and better forms of insulin, including insulin taken by nasal spray or by oral pill rather than by daily shots, will become a reality. Insulin by injection, however, will be given through a "closed loop" pump, meaning that a tiny detector will sense the body's blood sugar level and direct the pump to give out just the right amount of insulin, over time, to keep the blood sugar levels at a constant normal state.

In effect, it will act just like the pancreas itself, producing insulin on demand and the resulting good control of blood sugar will mean much less damage to the eyes, heart, kidneys, and the vessels of the legs. Better still, stem cells will allow a transplant to replace the ailing pancreas and in such a way that there will be no rejection and hence no antirejection drugs. Alternatively, stem cells will be placed in a microcontainer which will allow them to develop into islet cells, detect the level of blood sugar, and then release insulin without being attacked by the body's immune cells.

Organ transplants will be much safer and more effective as a result of much better antirejection drugs, which will result in better organ function, a longer, useful life of the transplanted organ, and fewer drug side effects. But as more and more people need a transplant and as the number of available organs remains steady, the waiting list will only grow and grow. Xenotransplantation, using organs from genetically modified animals such as pigs, will make hearts, kidneys, and other organs available on demand. No longer will you need to pray, in effect, for another person to die in order to save your own or a loved one's life nor will it be necessary for a relative to donate a kidney or part of a liver.

New approaches will prevent and treat that other major cause of death and disability: stroke. For example, we know that aneurysms begin to develop at an early age and only grow to the point of rupturing later in life. By looking at MRI scans, we will be able to determine which ones are potentially dangerous and which ones are irrelevant; the dangerous ones can be fixed by relatively noninvasive techniques such as the placement of platinum wires via a catheter or possibly by the use of ultrasound to coagulate and destroy the root of the aneurysm.

Neuroscience is advancing quickly. There is the potential to regenerate viable nerve activity damaged after stroke and trauma. And there will be ways to prevent further nerve and brain injury from trauma, disease, and strokes. We may soon have ways for the brain to tell an artificial limb to move. These are just some of the ways that will allow return of function and a continued useful life where no such hope has existed in the past.

There will be techniques to enter the arteries in the brain where the clot is located and not just dissolve it with tPA, but to actually retrieve it via a catheter. Risky to be sure, but worth the risk in certain situations. But preventing stroke is critical, and statins, those drugs used to reduce cholesterol and thereby reduce heart disease, have been shown to reduce strokes as well. Taking a pill is not the best medicine if it is not joined to a program of sound nutrition, exercise, and no smoking. It is very important for everyone to understand that the first evidence of a brain attack or stroke means get to the ER right away so that the appropriate steps can be taken to reverse the situation before irreversible damage sets in. Don't wait around to see if the speech problem or movement problem or inability to smile goes away. Time is of the essence.

Vaccines will be expanded to prevent ever more infections such as dengue, malaria, and tuberculosis. A vaccine for HIV seems far away, but it will come in time, although never soon enough. And now we have the first vaccines to prevent specific types of cancer: the hepatitis B vaccine to prevent liver cancer and the human papilloma virus vaccine to prevent cervical cancer. There will be many more such vaccines to prevent cancer, especially those known to be caused by infections, during the next five to fifteen years.

Remarkably, there will be vaccines for diseases not caused by infection—many chronic and disabling diseases will give way to a vaccine. There will be designer vaccines for treating individuals who have developed cancer. And to everyone's applause, vaccines will be administered not with needles but with patches, nasal sprays, pills, or other approaches.

Because we will be living longer, there will be a longer opportunity for body parts to wear out. I will give you some suggestions to slow that process, but medical science is working hard to give you repaired parts or new parts. Will it be like going to the auto repair shop and getting a new muffler after the old one wears out? Not quite. But do expect to see replacement organs, reconstructed tissues, heart valves that mimic the original, and better hip replacements that can be inserted with minimally invasive surgery.

And there will be repairs of knees that are worn out rather than being replaced as they are today. The new imaging equipment will show damage or stress to the knee lining very early, and this will allow for early therapy or preventive techniques to slow down the damage process. Perhaps your doctor can recommend special exercises or to avoid some activities. Or she may repair a subtle tear in the knee lining or insert new cells to create a new lining, making your knee seem years younger. In a sense, medicine will go beyond managing diseases to allowing the body to persist functionally for a much longer period of time than ever before. It is about not just dealing with the ravages of disease, but also dealing with the body parts that have worn out.

MORE THOUGHTS ABOUT THE FUTURE

These advances are transforming health care to its very core, and there is more to come. One of the changes that has happened and will continue to occur in medicine is a change from a male dominated profession to one where women are equal partners. When I was in medical school in the 1960s, fewer than 10 percent of students were women. Today it is about 50 percent. Back then women were encouraged to go into pediatrics, pathology or, if they really wanted to do surgery, then into obstetrics and gynecology. Today's residents in surgery are as likely to be women, and women now are chairs of surgical departments in major medical centers.

Some of what I have laid out in the preceding chapters are changes in medical care or the application of our current knowledge, translated from laboratory to clinical care. But many others are truly disruptive technologies—new concepts and new approaches that will impact how medical care is rendered.

Genomics certainly fits this category of a totally new approach, a new era that will have a major impact. Stem cells, should we learn how to use and manipulate them as scientists are predicting, will likewise profoundly impact and allow for the development of regenerative medicine. Dr. Richard Satava, a professor of surgery at the University of Washington in Seattle, and until recently leader of the Advanced Biomedical Technologies Program at the government's Defense Advanced Research Projects Agency (DARPA), speaks of the "biointelligence age" to indicate how new technologies will be converted from *dumb* to *intelligent*. Microchips and other technologies will be imbedded into inanimate objects and change them to "smart and active" objects.

Consider the automobile as an analogy. Today's automobile has more than fifty minicomputers that do everything from sensing the air in the tires to releasing the airbag to helping to navigate under difficult braking circumstances. So the automobile is no longer just a dumb machine that a human drives. It has actually become a highly interactive transportation system, which, in its way, interacts with a human driver.

We can think of RFID technology in somewhat the same sense. Recall our discussion of its use by Wal-Mart as part of their supply chain's inventory control systems. But let's take it another step. As described by Dr. Satava, Dr. Shankar Sastry at Berkeley coined the concept of *smart dust* in 1996. "A farmer plows the field and spreads the seeds, pesticide, and fertilizer along with billions of tiny smart computers the size of a pinhead—the RFIDs. Some are sensors and some are transmitters. As the plants grow, the RFIDs are incorporated into the plant to store information about the plant. When the harvesting machine comes along, the plants "talk" directly to the harvester—"pick me; my vegetable is ready"—determining those which are ripe as measured by the microsensors. As the vegetable is sent along the supply chain from farm to shipping to warehouse to grocery store, the information is continuously tracked. Then, when you go to the grocery store with your handheld computer such as a PDA or a souped-up cell phone, the vegetable will talk to your computer, telling how many calories, the shelf life, the price, and so forth. When you leave the store, all the contents in the shopping basket broadcast their information at the checkout counter, and you are automatically checked out."[1] Not only this, but if contamination is detected (ala the spinach that carried toxic E coli), the RFID tags will tell exactly from which farm and where on the farm the tainted food came.

If it can be done in the automobile and if it can be done, in principle at least, in agriculture, there is no reason why it cannot be done in medicine—and it will be.

ETHICS AND MEDICINE ARE NOT ALIGNED

Science is accelerating rapidly, and it will only continue to do so in the years ahead. Unfortunately, our social responses to the critical ethical issues raised by the new science have not kept pace. A national debate right now questions how we should approach stem cells, but it is unfortunately limited to simply the use or nonuse of embryonic stem cells. Lines are drawn, positions are rigid. Negotiations and meaningful discussions are minimal. But we need to be engaged in thoughtful and rational discussions, without hyperbole, of where and under what circumstances stem cells should be considered for use.

The same goes for our rapidly increasing knowledge of our own genes and what they can predict. Should we try to change them—to cure sickle cell anemia or cystic fibrosis? Should we try to change them to prevent diabetes mellitus in a person who is predisposed? Should we control whether we can have a boy or a girl baby? What about other genes the child could have—do we want to make use of our knowledge to decide our child's eye color, hair color, and stature? (I would venture to say this is interesting but trivial.)

What about trying to avoid the genes that might lead to an early death—a significant issue? Or since we know the genes from animals that can see well at night, do we want to add that gene to our child to allow them night vision? Then there are bigger questions, such as: How long should we live? When is long enough? This is turn leads to who should be able to get a transplanted organ? Is it simply a matter of whoever can pay for it can have it? If we could create suspended animation—which, by the way, is likely possible in the near future—would you think it appropriate to place a person in that state until a cure could be found for their currently lethal disease? If so, then who gets to choose? What would you do if you could come back younger than your great-great-grandchild?

I have discussed many new devices and potential devices that could be of great use in medicine. But who should get them, under what circumstances, and who will pay?

We truly need to start considering these sorts of issues because science will continue to move ahead. The question is, will we be ready?

PUBLIC HEALTH

As a country, the United States focuses on the individual, and so it is with medicine. We put a lot of emphasis into individual medical care but little into public health. Yet history has proven that addressing public health issues has a huge return for each individual. Consider that our teeth today are much better than in previous generations, not because we brush better, but because of universal fluoridation. In our system, the relatively well get all too little care, but the relatively ill get all too much. We have disparities among races, we have too high an infant mortality rate, and we have huge numbers of people with little or no insurance for catastrophic care needs.

Our health care system is great at dealing with acute episodes of disease, but not at longitudinal care. We spend 15 percent or so of our gross domestic product for health care, yet we have a population with unhealthy characteristics such as overweight, tobacco use, drug use, and lack of exercise. All of these will lead to higher health care costs later. For example, we know that any single blood sugar test that is over two hundred is a harbinger not only of diabetes, but also of many other problems the person's future, such as urinary tract infections, blood clots in the legs, heart disease, kidney disease, and many others.

In New York City, there is a new program run by the city health department that has each result of a specialized test for diabetes treatment routinely sent into the department. The department will then use public health techniques to assist those with problem results to manage their diabetes better. This could be money spent very well.

It is well known that diabetes in combination with heart failure is not only common, but that the rates of admissions to the hospital are much higher than with heart failure alone. Focusing on these patients can have a real impact on the individual's care and the total costs of the nation's health care. One approach used by some managed care companies is to have case managers follow these patients and monitor their diabetes and their heart failure with simple phone calls on a regular basis, and for the patients to use electronic devices that send in their weight and blood sugar to the case manager daily. If these start to vary, the nurse can immediately contact the patient and change medications, for example, as needed.

The result is many fewer admissions to the hospital. Good for the patient and good for the overall cost of care. But generally, our system of care does not have the proper incentives to encourage this approach. I predict that we will change—and soon. Not because it is better medicine, which it is, but because it will save the insurers, including the federal government, a lot of money.

The same goes for vaccines. As I said in the vaccine chapter, other than lifestyle factors, the least expensive and most effective way to prevent many diseases is through the use of vaccines. Certainly this has proven true for many, many infectious diseases that used to ravage society—and still do in the developing world. But in the future, we can expect to see vaccines make a profound difference for many noninfectious diseases as well, including cancer, diabetes, arthritis, and possibly heart disease. Here again, vaccination is money well spent. But will we vaccinate our daughters to prevent cervical cancer? Will we get the vaccine to prevent shingles? And will our tort system be adjusted to encourage the pharmaceutical firms to actively engage in vaccine research and marketing again?

AGING GRACEFULLY—FOR A LONG TIME

My message throughout this book is that a series of megatrends will revolutionize medical care for you, your children, and your grandchildren. Remarkable advances have the potential to create longer, healthier lives. But my internist likes to remind me that no matter how much we can extend life, we will still die. Most of us will experience some type of illness, acute or chronic, on the way out. So despite all the vast improvements in medical care, which each of us can and will benefit from, disease still lies ahead. As the population ages certain diseases are more prevalent. I worry about how little has been done so far by medical scientists to deal with some of these, and how little most of us do as individuals to deal with others. Here are a few things that worry me a lot.

First, there is little on the horizon that I can see to slow the process of Alzheimer's disease. As we become an aged population, dementia will prevail in our society. Certainly a lot of research is ongoing in this field, but right now there is little to show for it in terms of actually treating or preventing Alzheimer's. There are some drugs available of limited value, and vaccines are being studied. But until there are some breakthroughs, we will see large numbers of us suffering from dementia and being burdens to ourselves, our children, and society as a whole.

Second, we all need to realize that a natural aging process affects our bodies. A good rule of thumb is that we lose about 1 percent per year of many of our functions, such as lung function, kidney function, or bone strength. We can skip having birthday parties, but we cannot avoid the fact that we are going to get older each year, each month, and each day. So what can we do? While we cannot slow the march of time, we can slow the aging process. But I worry that most of us don't find the time or energy to help our bodies be what they could or should be. Here are some suggestions and most of them relate to exercise, nutrition, and stress management.

There are hints—although not real proof yet—that we can slow the onset of Alzheimer's disease with mental exercise—active mental exercise. Sitting in front of the television does not count, but doing crossword puzzles, playing chess, or the new numbers craze, Sudoku, do count, as does staying mentally engaged by interacting with friends. The worst thing is to be cooped up alone in your home for much of the day during your elder years. Yes, the old home has wonderful memories, but it is much better to move to an active retirement community where, even if your mobility is limited, multiple ongoing activities engage your mind.

Studies also show that regular church attendance adds to longevity. Maybe it is the religious experience, maybe it's the attendant meditation inherent in many church routines, but probably it is also the result of being engaged with others. So keep your mind active; give it regular exercise. Physical exercise is important as well, perhaps because it keeps the blood flowing, and sound nutrition is key. New data suggest that a diet that is good for your heart is also good for your brain. Just as the omega-3 fatty acids (DHA and ARA) help your baby's brain to develop, they also seem to help slow the onset of age-related dementia.

What about those organs that are losing 1 percent of their function each year? Let's use our bones as an example of what you can do to help yourself. At birth our bones have little calcium in them, but as we grow and mature, calcium and other minerals are laid down to create strength. Our *bone mineral density* (BMD) reaches its peak between the ages of eighteen and twenty-four. The peak level each of us reaches depends upon whether we ate enough high-calcium foods during the first twenty years of our life, and if we exercised regularly to help create the environment for the minerals to be laid down in the bone. But after our early twenties, we cannot increase our bone mineral density further. It is done.

It stops at that level and stays there until about age thirty-five, at which time we start to lose about 1 percent of our bone mineral density per year. So by the time we reach eighty-five or ninety-five, we have lost quite a lot and the risk of a fracture if we fall is greatly increased. For women, the rate of loss markedly increases with menopause and continues at that higher rate for about five years; then it settles back to the 1 percent loss per year. But that extra loss for those five or so years means that women reach a point of easy fractures (osteoporosis) sooner than men do. And since women on average live longer than men, there are ultimately more women with osteoporosis in the elder population, and hence we tend to see more women having fractures. But as both men and women live longer we are also going see more men with fractured bones in their elder years.

You can slow the loss of minerals from your bones. Watch your calcium and vitamin D intake. Most Americans do not get enough calcium in their diets as adults, so a supplement may be needed. Because we tend to work in office buildings rather than on the farm, we do not get enough sunlight to keep our vitamin D levels up, so another supplement is needed by most older adults, especially in the winter months.

Bone strength depends on bone use, so exercise is important as well. Simple walking—regularly—puts appropriate stress on the leg, hip, and backbones. But, I know, you work all day, and it's dark when you get home, so you cannot walk. Well, then, do it in small doses during the day; avoid the elevator, walk to meetings, use the staircase. It can add up quickly.

Just because you pop some calcium citrate tablets and a vitamin D pill does not mean you should not eat a diet rich in these vitamins and minerals—like whole grains and dark green leafy vegetables. We have been taught to like iceberg lettuce, which has little or no nutritional value, in our salads instead of eating greens like arugula, dandelion, or spinach. We have been trained to eat white bread and white rice rather than whole wheat, brown rice, oatmeal, or barley. Try them. After a while, you will not want to go back, and you will have done a good deed for your bone strength and your health in general.

What about other organs like the heart and lungs? Exercise is key. Aerobic exercise (walking, running, swimming, biking) pushes the heart to work harder—which it likes. How hard should you exercise? A simple rule of thumb is to go for a level of exercise that makes you break out in a light sweat and keep it up for twenty to thirty minutes, three or more times each week. You will feel the difference, and you will like how you feel.

Also do some weight-bearing exercises like those of Nautilus machines. Get some help when you start to pick out exercise machines for your legs, hips, torso, and arms, and get advice on how much weight and how many repetitions to do.

In addition to exercise, you need sound nutrition. Despite the competing claims, the basics are straightforward. Eat whole grains (whole wheat, not white bread; brown, not white rice), fresh vegetables cooked at home in a way to preserve their goodness (stir fried or steamed, but not boiled), and lots of fruits. Limit meat and choose low-fat cuts. Do eat fresh fish and use monosaturated oils to cook (olive oil); in both cases, the oils are actually good for you in reasonable amounts. Avoid prepared foods; cook from scratch. It really does not have to take much longer to prepare, and the taste will be much, much better. And then, if you really follow this approach, it's okay to treat yourself occasionally with a few potato chips or a chocolate chip cookie.

The brain, just like other organs, ages with time. It, too, probably reaches its peak at about age twenty, so you need to stimulate your children and grandchildren to pursue intellectual activities during the growing years. It's like creating a functional reserve in the brain. Then keep using it, and it will stay much healthier. People who continue to make intellectual use of their brains into retirement will have better success holding off dementia. And this, too, can be helped with physical exercise and sound nutrition.

The good news: You will feel a lot better; your heart, lungs, and kidneys will be happier; and your muscles will retain their strength. And your brain will keep working much longer. So instead of losing 1 percent function per year you can actually slow it way down—not to zero—but way down. Modest exercise, three times each week, has been shown to reduce cardiovascular deaths by 50 percent! And it also reduces cancer. We do age, and we will die. But we can put it off and keep our bodies working well for a long time.

A third concern that I have is that many people still smoke, and many teens are starting to smoke. Smoking ruins your lungs, sets you up for many different cancers, and is bad for your heart. Tobacco is one of the hardest addictions to overcome, but you can do it, and there are programs and medications that can help. Don't delay.

I really worry that we, as a society and as individuals, do not address stress—and our lives are full of it. Jobs, child rearing, and family issues all create stress, and we need to find constructive ways to reduce it. We cannot avoid stress; it is all around us, so we need to confront it and find ways to reduce and control it. Appropriate nonjudgmental discussion can help. Exercise helps by burning up some of the stress-induced chemicals that make us feel bad. Meditation can help as well. Remember the discussion about PET scans and functional MRI? Those same imaging techniques have been used to study meditation. Real changes occur in the brain with meditation, and individuals who regularly meditate experience greater changes. Like exercise and a good diet—once you try it, I predict you will like it.

Finally, I am also concerned that we are raising children today who will be set up for health problems in later years. Remember that the peak bone mineral density is reached at about age twenty. Same for their muscles, brains, and all other organs. From then on it's too late to add more; it's all downhill. So make sure that your kids and grandkids get the nutrients and the exercise that they need to build those strong bones now. Teenagers don't get enough exercise, and they need it. Our use of prepared foods, including soft drinks, means that the calcium and mineral input is often way lacking.

A well-exercised brain during childhood is like making stronger bones. We really can add to our capabilities during youth. But once the brain development is done, then it's done. It's downhill from there, although a lifetime of mental exercise slows that decay as well. So do your kids a favor, and be sure that they really challenge their brains—not just sit in front of the TV. The important point is that what we do as parents and grandparents to assist our kids grow and develop will markedly affect how they will enjoy health or be beset with chronic illnesses decades and decades later.

AGING SUCCESSFULLY

To some degree I have already dealt with this issue, but here is a summary based on the suggestions of noted gerontologists. Before birth, you would do well to choose long-lived parents; have your mother get good, regular prenatal care, have your mother not smoke or drink alcohol; and have your mother take prenatal vitamins. From birth to age sixty, you should exercise regularly, remain lean, get enough calcium in your diet, wear your seatbelt, get regular medical exams and vaccinations, not smoke, drink in moderation, avoid violence and illicit drugs, practice safe sex, and have a successful marriage.

When you reach age sixty, keep up the good work, but add exercise if you don't exercise regularly and include balance exercises (so you won't trip and break a leg); maintain a steady weight (assuming you are not obese); avoid taking any unnecessary meds; and have regular mental activity, socialization, and intellectual inputs. And then when you reach age eighty, do all of the former things, but also safety proof your home to avoid falls, use a cane to prevent falls if you are unsteady—it's no time for being brave—and keep on doing whatever it is that you have been doing because it has worked so far.[2]

RECAP

To recap, medical care is in the process of a revolution, actually multiple revolutions that are reflecting and will continue to reflect—for the better—your care into the future. Research into genomics will have major implications for disease prediction, prevention, diagnosis, and treatment. Stem cells hold out the promise of organ repair and regeneration. Advances in imaging are allowing us to see deep into the body, creating remarkable pictures of anatomy, and increasingly telling us of the body's functions, right down to the cellular level.

Engineers are developing powerful devices—many of them remarkably small—that can assist our bodies when broken or damaged. The possibility of replacement organs like hearts and kidneys transplanted from animals is no longer far-fetched. Surgery is changing dramatically with less invasive surgery, much better preoperative information, and lots that can be done without the need for an actual surgical procedure, such as inserting a graft inside the aorta to cure a large aneurysm. Simulators and robotics will make surgery more accurate and much safer.

Medical information is increasingly being digitized so that your medical record can either go everywhere with you or can be accessed anywhere via the Internet. Preventable medical errors can be attacked and dramatically reduced. And we can benefit from the ancient wisdoms of other cultures and times with complementary medicine techniques such as acupuncture, meditation, massage—and we can benefit from prayer.

We can put all these advances to our benefit to help prevent illness and to treat it when it occurs. But it is equally important that we do take good care of the body we have been entrusted with. That is our own personal obligation. No doctor or nurse or procedure or pill can do that for us. So in closing, let me ask you to imagine if the following person sounds in any way like you.

COULD THIS BE YOU?

You have a good job. You have done well at it, and you can see the opportunities for promotion in the years to come. But it is hard work, requires lots of hours, and lots of stress. You have a nice family whom you love dearly, but you have relatively little time with them. You are overweight—not obese—but you know it would be good to lose ten to twenty pounds. You know you do not get enough exercise, so you actually bought a membership to a health club about six months ago, but cannot quite remember the last time you went.

In the morning, you need to get to work early, so you skip breakfast and stop for a mocha latte and a blueberry scone to eat in the car while driving to work. Lunch will be something picked up from a fast-food outlet and possibly even eaten at your desk. There will be no time to cook dinner, so you will, once more, get carry-out. You know it would be nice to have the whole family sit down together for dinner, but that is just not practical and besides, right after supper you need to go pick up your older child who will have just finished soccer practice. You are thinking that there is not enough time with your family. Perhaps this weekend . . . but not until you make some progress on that big presentation that you will be making on Monday morning.

Does this sound like you—even a little like you? The simple fact is that it sounds like many of us. If it is you, I hate to say it, but the fact is that you are a disaster waiting to happen. The good news is, now you know it, and so you can do something about it.

You *can* make a difference. Your body will love you for it. It is not hard, but it does take some time—each and every day. Enjoy your health in the knowledge that if you keep your body and mind at peak performance, then the fruits of the new megatrends in medicine, with the help of your health care providers, will be able to make remarkable inroads in preventing illness or, indeed, return you to health if you are injured or develop a serious disease.

This book has been about the megatrends that are rapidly changing medical practice and will continue to do so into the foreseeable future. But it is equally about how you need to be responsible for your own health—actually not all that hard to do. But our society is such today that it seems difficult—hard to find whole grain bread, hard to find time to exercise, hard to find time with our families, hard to deal with the stresses of ordinary life. But in order to be and remain healthy, you really need to address these issues and not use them as excuses.

If you do confront them head-on, then you can likely enjoy a long and productive life and be well situated to benefit from the remarkable progress that is occurring in medicine today.

Notes

Introduction

1. Lewis Thomas, MD, then chancellor of the Memorial Sloan Kettering Cancer Center in New York City, wrote a wonderful small book in 1983 called *The Youngest Science: Notes of a Medicine-Watcher*, published by Viking Press. In this book he described his own career spanning the 1930s and onward and how he observed (and was very much a part of) these major changes toward medicine becoming a science.

Chapter 1

1. Throughout this book I have not only changed patients' names but have made other substantive changes to their history to ensure that they cannot be identified. However, the essence of their stories is true.

2. RNA is comprised of a sugar-phosphate backbone with four nucleotides, like DNA; but instead of thymine (T), it substitutes uracil (U).

3. An excellent, albeit scientific, review of some of the implications of pharmacogenomics is in an article by W.E. Evans and H. L. McLeod, *New England Journal of Medicine* 348 (2003): 538-549.

4. dihydropyrimidine dehydrogenase.

5. ApoE4 is also associated with an increased risk for late onset Alzheimer's disease developing after age sixty to sixty-five. Having two copies of apoE4 further increases that risk. It is a risk factor, however, not a cause, and not everyone who has apoE4 goes on to develop Alzheimer's—just as many people with Alzheimer's have apoE3 or 2.

6. A. Finch et al., *Journal of the American Medical Association* 296 (2006):185–192.

7. A good recent study of genomic signatures in breast cancer is by Fan et al. in the *New England Journal of Medicine* 355 (2006): 560–569. This was accompanied by an editorial by J. O'Shaughnessy, *NEJM* 355 (2006): 615–617. The study showed that it is possible with microarray molecular signatures to separate those who have and do not have a good prognosis. The editorial emphasized that biologic activity of a tumor is more important than simple anatomy in prediction of outcomes. In the same issue was a paper by Potti, et al. that showed similar results in separating high risk of recurrence from low risk among those with early stage lung cancer. *NEJM* 355 (2006): 570–580.

8. L Bullinger et al,. *New England Journal of Medicine* 350 (2004): 1605-1616.

9. A Rosenwald A et al., *New England Journal of Medicine* 346 (2002): 1937-1947.

10. National Institutes of Health (www.nih.gov). This will take you to the Home Page, where there are pages for researchers and pages for patients and their families. They are easy to follow. Be aware that the NIH is careful to only advocate drugs, procedure or approaches that have been well proven to be effective.

Chapter 2

1. It is actually a very complicated process. Briefly described, the cells are placed in petri dishes that have a lining across the bottom made up of cells from a mouse embryo. Somehow these cells are critical, probably by producing a set of chemicals that help direct the growth of the stem cells. To this dish are added fluids with nutrients. Each day the nutrients must be replenished. Once a week the growing colony of stem cells must be split into two or more new dishes; otherwise they will be overcrowded. Every two weeks, they need a new layer of mouse feeder cells. Then the next steps are performed. The stem cells now need to be induced to develop into the cell type desired—islet cells, brain cells, heart cells, etc. A lot of steps and a lot still to learn.
2. N. Dib et al., *Circulation Journal of the American Heart Association* 112 (2005): 1748–1755.
3. C. Steinwender et al., *American Heart Journal* 151(6) (2006):1296.e7–1296.e13.
4. In medical trials, we like to do controlled studies. The idea is to compare a new treatment versus an older treatment—Drug A in one group of patients versus Drug B in another group of patients. Or injection of stem cells in some patients versus no injection in other patients. Generally, we like to do randomized studies, meaning that patients are randomly allocated to Drug A or Drug B, or to receive stem cells or not. Finally, the most powerful studies are those that are "blind." This means that neither doctor nor patient knows which treatment patients received. In this way, the patient will not "feel better" because they thought that the treatment should work. Similarly, the doctor will not "over read" positive results just because he or she was certain that the new treatment ought to work.
5. L. E. Wold et al., 204; 10:294–301. This paper, written for professionals, is fairly easy to read and, although a few years old, offers a good overview of directions in this field.
6. The five studies mentioned are reviewed in an editorial in the *New England Journal of Medicine*, by Dr A. Rosenzweig of the Beth Israel–Deaconess Hospital, Boston and the Harvard Stem Cell Institute. *NEJM* 355 (2006): 1274–1277.
7. A good discussion of cancer stem cells can be found in an article by Craig Jordan, Monica Guzman, and Mark Noble of the University of Rochester. *NEJM* 355 (2006): 1253–1260.

Chapter 3

1. A. A. Parker, *New England Journal of Medicine* 335 (2006): 447–455.
2. M. N. Oxman et al., *New England Journal of Medicine* 353 (2005): 2271–2284.
3. Y. Okura et al., *Proceedings of the National Academy of Sciences USA* 103 (2006): 9619–9624.
4. If you are concerned, I suggest that you have a thorough discussion with your pediatrician and perhaps check out these two Web sites (www.aap.org/parents [American Academy of Pediatrics] and www.immunizationinfo.org/immunizationissues [National Network for Immunization Information])
5. Henschle, C.L., et al, *New England Journal of Medicine* 355 (2006): 1763-71.

Chapter 4

1. An angiogram involves inserting a catheter into the big artery in the groin, advancing it up into the arteries of the heart and then injecting a substance that will show up on the X-ray.

The next step is to take a film of the blood flow through the coronary arteries with the X-ray equipment. Today these films are very detailed and accurate.

2. Henschle, C.L., et al., *New England journal of Medicine* 355 (2006): 1763-71.

Chapter 5

1. As I have suggested elsewhere, look only to reputable Web sites beginning with the National Institutes of Health (www.nih.gov), those of major academic medical centers, or large national health organizations such as the American Heart Association, the American Cancer Society, or the Juvenile Diabetes Society, to name a few.

Chapter 6

1. About 350,000 Americans are on dialysis today, with about 75,000 on a kidney transplant waiting list. But only about 15,000 transplants get done each year because of the dearth of supply. The situation will only get worse as the epidemic of diabetes produces more individuals with end-stage kidney disease. By 2010 it is estimated that some 600,000–800,000 people will be on dialysis, but the number of transplants will be about the same.

Chapter 7

1. From an interview by F. Irving, "Mission: EHR," *Advance for Health Information Executives* (2005 April), 21–28.
2. You might look for Web sites that abide by the TRUSTe code of conduct. TRUSTe is a nonprofit enabling trust based on privacy for personal information on the Internet. See www.truste.org.

Chapter 8

1. See T. Bodenheimer, *Annals of Internal Medicine* 142 (2005): 932–937, for a good discussion of the relation of technologic innovation and rising health care costs.
2. D. M. Cutler, A. B. Rosen, and S. Vijan, *New England Journal of Medicine*, 355 (2006): 920–927.

Chapter 9

1. D. Eisenberg et al., *New England Journal of Medicine* 328 (1993): 246–252.
2. B. M. Berman et al., *Annals of Internal Medicine*, 141 (2004): 901–910.
3. P. White et al., *Annals of Internal Medicine* 141 (2004): 911–918.
4. M. M. Beckmann, Cochrane Database System Rev, 2006;[1]: CD005123 and *Journal of the American Med Association* 295 (2006): 1361-1362.
5. S. E. Straus, *New England Journal of Medicine* 347 (Year?): 1997-1998.
6. Bill Moyers, *Healing and the Mind* (Doubleday, New York: Doubleday, 1993).
7. For a good description of meditation go to the National Center for Alternative and Complementary Medicine Web site, www.nccam.nih.gov.
8. A. Lutz, et al., *Proceedings of the National Academy of the Sciences* 101 (2004): 16369-16373.
9. Shingles is caused by the same virus that causes chicken pox. After infection with chicken pox, the virus lives in the body in a latent stage, but then can break out at a time of low immunity, such as with aging or radiation for cancer. A vaccine to prevent shingles in the elderly has recently been approved by the FDA. (See the chapter on vaccines.)

10. Herbert Benson, *The Relaxation Response* (New York: William Morrow, 1975).
11. D. Spiegel et al., *Lancet* 2 (1989): 888–891.
12. M. A. Richardson, et al., *Alternative Therapies in Health and Medicine* 3 (1997): 62-70.
13. R. C. Byrd, *Southern Medical Journal* 81 (1988):826–829.
14. W. S. Harris, *Archives of Internal Medicine* 159 (1999): 2273-2278.
15. L. Dossey, *Healing Words: The Power of Prayer* (New York: HapperCollins, 1993).
16. H. Benson et al., *American Heart Journal* 151 (2006): 934–942.
17. Dean Ornish, *Reversing Heart Disease,* (New York: Ballentine Books, 1990).
18. D. T. Stern and M. Papadakis, "The Developing Physician—Becoming a Professional" *New England Journal of Medicine* 355 (2006): 1794-1799.

Chapter 10

1. Leape, L. et al., *New England Journal of Medicine* 1991, 324: 377–384.
2. Andrews, L. et al., *The Lancet,* 1997, 349: 309–313.
3. Clinical Initiatives Center, "First Do No Harm," 6–7, The Advisory Board Company, Washington, D.C., (2000).
4. L. T. Kohn, J. M. Corrigan, and M. S. Donaldson, for the Institute of Medicine, "To Err is Human: Building a Safer Health Care System" (Washington, D.C: National Academy Press 1999).
5. L. L. Leape, D. M. Berwick, "Five years after To Err is Human: what have we learned?" *Journal of the American Medical Association* 293 (2005): 2384–90.
6. G. J. Annas, "The Patient's Right to Safety: Improving the Quality of Care through Litigation against Hospitals," *New England Journal of Medicine* 354 (2006): 2063–2066.
7. Angela Stephan, Stephen and Associates, personal communication, 2006 May.
8. R. Amalberti, Y. Auroy, D. Berwick, and P. Barach, "Five System Barriers to Achieving Ultrasafe Health Care," *Annals Internal Medicine* 142 (2005): 756–764.
9. Pramrod Raheja, personal communication, Human Performance Training Institute and pilot for United Airlines, 2006 January.
10. For more on simulators and robotics, see the chapter on the OR of the Future.

Chapter 11

1. Richard Satava, MD, personal communication, 2006.
2. Adapted from a presentation by Les Katzel, MD, PhD, 2004 October.

Acknowledgments

First and foremost, I owe a real debt of gratitude to all of those who willingly spent their time to teach me about their areas of expertise and to help me synthesize these thoughts into concepts. Since there were so many, I cannot thank each of them by name, but I am truly grateful. I will give special mention to all of those at the Telemedicine and Advanced Technology Research Center of the Army for allowing me access to many of their meetings. Also, Richard Satava, MD, formerly of the Defense Advanced Research Projects Agency, and John Gallin, MD, the Director of the Clinical Center of the National Institutes of Health. Each not only gave of his time, but offered suggestions and access to many others.

Joanne Kaback helped me to convert my initial medical thoughts into a more lay-person friendly writing style. Brian Hampton, Vice President and Associate Publisher at Thomas Nelson, encouraged me to dictate each chapter as though I were giving a talk to a lay group. His suggestion helped me avoid getting too scientific. Margaret Frazier took my dictated tapes and turned them into the first drafts of chapters. Nancy Jackson, a copy editor at the *Baltimore Sun,* corrected my grammar and made each chapter much easier to read.

Colleagues who reviewed individual chapters for me included Barry Meisenberg, MD, George Ludwig, MD, Carol Tackett, MD, Michael Minear, Dennis Duda, Reuben Mezrich, MD, PhD, David Berkowitz, Brian Berman, MD, James Kagan, Warren Grundfest, MD, PhD and Gerald Moses, PhD. Thanks are also due to Tom Jemski along with Sonia Garcia for assistance with the graphics.

The professionals at Thomas Nelson were not only supportive but eager to help. Paula Major, Bryan Norman, Geoff Stone, and freelancer Janene Macivor made the work fun while helping me to be clear, concise, and complete.

Our daughter, Becky, gave me excellent advice on what readers would want to know and want to do as a result of reading each section, and our son-in-law, Brian Kushnir, organized a brainstorming session to think out the directions of the book. And of special note, my wife, Carol, was not only always supportive, but also made sure I had the time for interviews, reading, and writing.